T0258587

Encyclopedia of Coronary Artery Disease: Integrated Therapies

Volume IV

Encyclopedia of Coronary Artery Disease: Integrated Therapies
Volume IV

Edited by **Warren Lyde**

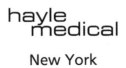

hayle
medical

New York

Published by Hayle Medical,
30 West, 37th Street, Suite 612,
New York, NY 10018, USA
www.haylemedical.com

Encyclopedia of Coronary Artery Disease: Integrated Therapies
Volume IV
Edited by Warren Lyde

International Standard Book Number: 978-1-63241-141-9 (Hardback)

Printed in the United States of America.

Contents

Preface

In my initial years as a student, I used to run to the library at every possible instance to grab a book and learn something new. Books were my primary source of knowledge and I would not have come such a long way without all that I learnt from them. Thus, when I was approached to edit this book; I became understandably nostalgic. It was an absolute honor to be considered worthy of guiding the current generation as well as those to come. I put all my knowledge and hard work into making this book most beneficial for its readers.

The death rate due to ischemic heart disease has declined in current years. The improved comprehension of risk factors related to the growth of coronary artery disease has considerably contributed to this decrease. Enhancements in medical and interventional therapy have minimized the problems related to acute myocardial infection as well as revascularization. After the introduction of imaging methodologies, the noninvasive characterization of regional function, metabolism and perfusion enabled more advanced tissue characterization to recognize changeable dysfunction with great prognostic and diagnostic accuracy. It can now be authentically claimed that computed tomography angiography (CTA) of the coronary arteries is available. In the examination of patients with suspected coronary artery disease, several guidelines today deem CTA as an alternative to stress testing. The nuclear method most commonly employed by cardiologists is myocardial perfusion imaging (MPI). The organization of CTA with a nuclear camera supports the achievement of cardiac function, coronary anatomy and MPI from a single piece of equipment. Evaluating cardiac viability is now quite ordinary with these optimizations to cardiac imaging. Conventional coronary angiography displays a variety of restraints associated with content, patient safety, image acquisition and interpretation. Obstacles to such enhancements consist of the lack of clinical outcomes studies associated with novel imaging technology, the requirement for physicians, staff member training, and the costs related to acquiring and efficiently using these enhancements in coronary angiography. This book contains significant information that each and every cardiologist needs to know. It contains two sections on coronary heart disease and noninvasive diagnostic approach in coronary heart disease.

I wish to thank my publisher for supporting me at every step. I would also like to thank all the authors who have contributed their researches in this book. I hope this book will be a valuable contribution to the progress of the field.

Editor

Something About Prevence of Coronary Heart Disease

Relationship Between Ox–LDL, Immune Cells, Atheroma Dimensions and Angiographic Measurements Assessed by Coronary Angiography and Intravascular Ultrasound

Catarina Ramos, Patrícia Napoleão,
Rui Cruz Ferreira, Cristina Fondinho, Mafalda Selas,
Miguel Mota Carmo, Ana Maria Crespo and
Teresa Pinheiro

Additional information is available at the end of the chapter

1. Introduction

In this chapter we report on the relationship between angiographic findings, measured by coronary angiography (CA) and intravascular ultrasound virtual histology (IVUS-VH) modalities, and indicators of vascular inflammation in the context of coronary artery disease (CAD). We sought to explore *in vivo* the relationship between patient demographics, anthropometric measures, risk factors, soluble biomarkers and plaque composition or its morphological characteristics.

The interplay of inflammatory cells, cytokines and indicators of cell death may concur to the plaque phenotype in the context of coronary artery disease. Therefore, the lymphocyte populations expressing CD4 and CD8, the circulating levels of oxidized low density lipoprotein (ox-LDL), which may be primarily originated in the atheroma, the levels of tumour necrosis factor alpha (TNF- α) and of soluble Fas ligand (sFasL), which may reflect the inflammatory response and vascular apoptosis, were studied.

These biomarkers would provide useful tools to improve medical diagnosis of the clinical atheroma. Noninvasive identification of high-risk/vulnerable coronary atherosclerotic plaques is one of the ultimate goals of coronary imaging and would dramatically improve risk stratification of both symptomatic and asymptomatic patients [1]. Therefore, correlations between plaque composition, bio-indicators and the severity of cardiac events may provide unique information about plaque type to enhance the precision of clinical and laboratory variables used to assess patients at risk of CAD.

1.1. Coronary artery disease

Coronary artery disease is still the main cause of death worldwide and coronary atherothrombosis is the leading cause of death in the United States and Europe [2,3]. A large number of individuals who die suddenly of CAD due to atherosclerosis have no previous symptoms [4].

Atherosclerosis is a chronic pathological process of the vasculature characterized by focal arterial wall inflammation that leads to plaque build-up, intraluminal narrowing, and atherothrombotic stenosis or occlusion with distal organ damage [5,6]. The atherosclerotic lesion is a thickening of the artery intima that consists of inflammatory and smooth muscle cells [7], as well as connective-tissue, lipids and debris [8]. The atheroma formation is initiated by an accumulation of lipid-laden cells beneath the endothelium, denominated fatty streak [9,10]. As atherosclerosis progresses from a benign phenotype, the atheroma becomes fibrotic, with a large necrotic core. Also, the plaque becomes more inflamed, resulting in an infiltration of macrophages and T-lymphocytes to the metabolically active fibrous cap [3]. Disintegration of foam cells and production of matrix metalloproteinases by activated leukocytes have detrimental consequences leading to the destabilization of lipid rich cores and the thinning of the fibrous cap [8]. This leads to a rupture-prone thin-cap fibroatheroma. The plaque rupture may cause arterial thrombosis, which results in a clinical spectrum of presentations ranging from sudden cardiac death, due to coronary occlusion, to an asymptomatic event with plaque progression [3]. In fact, the rupture of vulnerable atherosclerotic plaque is the cause of most acute coronary syndromes, e.g. myocardial infarction and unstable angina [8,11].

Atherosclerotic plaque stability is related to histological composition however biomarkers for the disease severity are still lacking today [12-14]. Multiple evidences link risk factors for atherosclerosis and its complications with altered histology, including the operation of both innate and adaptive immunity and the balance of stimulatory and inhibitory pathways that regulate their participation in atheroma formation and complication [15].

The early involvement of monocytes and macrophages in atherosclerosis is initiated with endothelial cell activation. Several protein mediators, specifically cytokines and chemokines, and LDL oxidative modification [16], direct monocyte migration to the intima and promote their maturation into macrophages, which are retained in the lesion [17,18]. These pro-inflammatory monocytes propagate the innate response by expressing high levels of pro-inflammatory cytokines and other macrophages mediators including metalloproteinases [6,19,20]. Dendritic cells that populate atherosclerotic plaques can present antigens to T-cells, which mount a cellular immune response [21]. These immune cells are also involved in thrombosis. Coagulation proteins elicit the expression of pro-inflammatory cytokines and mediators that interact with toll-like receptors of immune cells. These events promote endothelial cell apoptosis [22,23].

The ox-LDL has been described as a relevant pro-atherogenic autoantigen and its inflammatory and immunogenic activity has been implicated in atherosclerosis development and CAD [14,24]. Experimental data showed that ox-LDL is formed in the arterial wall where it is internalized by macrophages to form foam cells, contributing to the plaque progression [14]. The co-localization of ox-LDL with lymphocytes and monocyte-derived cells in the human atherosclerotic lesions reinforce the pro-atherogenic and immunogenic properties of ox-LDL, which was verified *in vitro* [24]. Eventually, ox-LDL formed in the arterial wall is released in the circulation [13], being their circulating levels strongly associated with angiographically documented coronary artery disease [25]. The proximity of ox-LDL and inflammatory cells, such as lymphocyte populations, in the atherosclerotic plaque may accelerate macrophage activity and therefore promote atherogenesis [26]. The T-cells expressing CD4 surface marker recognize antigens presented by dendritic cells and macrophages. The T-cell expressing CD8 when activated are capable of killing smooth muscle cells and macrophages. Both CD4 and CD8 T cells share the capacity to recognize protein antigens bound to histocompatibility molecules on cell surfaces [27].

Thus, the *in vivo* identification of plaque vulnerability whether by characterizing its components or by providing measures of plaque-related oxidative and inflammation markers may improve diagnostic and eventually allow the detection of vulnerable atheroma before rupture.

1.2. Coronary angiography

Since its implementation over 30 years ago, invasive coronary angiography has become the standard clinical method for describing the coronary arteries and the "gold standard" for diagnosing CAD. The use of contrast-enhanced coronary angiography has been introduced for stenosis detection and for assessing blood flow in the epicardial arteries. The approach based on edge-detection algorithms has also been proposed as an emerging tool for the detection, characterization, and quantification of coronary atherosclerotic plaques [11].

The increased understanding of atherosclerosis has highlighted inherent limitations of coronary angiography as a technique for the assessment of coronary atherosclerotic plaques. Angiography provides a 2-dimensional view of the arterial lumen, but with no visualization of the vessel wall. Atherosclerosis primarily affects the arterial wall and since only the lumen is displayed, angiography does not provide extensive information about the plaque [28,29] and may obscure the true plaque burden, leading to an underestimation of plaque severity [3]. Also, the atherosclerotic plaque initially grows in an outwardly manner, expanding to the vessel wall, a process denominated positive remodeling. Therefore, as a result of positive remodeling, angiography frequently fails to detect the early stages of atherosclerosis. Although positively remodeled lesions do not restrict blood flow, they may be unstable and may contribute to the onset of acute coronary syndromes [30]. Furthermore, because putative sites of stenosis are compared with an apparently normal arterial segment, angiography often fails to detect diffuse disease in which a large portion of the artery is impacted by atherosclerotic disease. Both positive remodeling and diffuse disease are common in atherosclerotic progression and may be determinants of clinical outcome.

Also, the assessment of angiograms is solely visual and, consequently, subject to significant variation in image interpretation (observer bias) which may lead to a significant underestimation of lesion severity [30].

Assessing the atheroma dimensions by coronary angiography (CA) has been more recently surpassed by new methods for cardiovascular imaging using ultrasound [28,29,31] and multislice CT [32-34], which allow a more accurate and complete imaging of atherosclerotic coronary vessels.

1.3. Intravascular ultrasound

Intravascular ultrasound (IVUS), a catheter-based technique that provides high resolution cross-sectional images of the coronary vessel in vivo, is a tomographic technique that permits two-dimensional visualization of the arterial wall and allows further characterization of its individual layers. Thus, IVUS is a unique imaging modality for the direct examination of vessel dimensions and arterial wall characteristics in live subjects.

The coronary artery is inspected by a catheter incorporating a miniature ultrasound transducer, which emits high-frequency ultrasound, usually in the range of 20 to 50 MHz providing an axial resolution of about 100–200 μm. Lateral resolution of the ultrasonic waves is less specific and may vary depending on imaging depth and beam width, averaging around 250 μm [35].

Given their proximity to the plaque, intravascular catheters have the inherent advantage of a high signal-to-noise ratio [3]. The information obtained through IVUS imaging depicts the morphological characteristics of the atheromatous plaque and is used to illustrate the geometrical configuration of its layers and architecture. Most clinical centers use a pullback system to withdraw the catheter at a constant rate of 0.5 mm/s following its initial deployment distal to the area of interest. As the transducer is moved through the artery, ultrasonic reflections are electronically converted to cross-sectional images [31]. This IVUS modality is called "virtual histology" IVUS (IVUS-VH) and allows the identification of the composition of atherosclerotic plaques by discriminating varying echolucent regions within the atheroma [12]. Four plaque components, fibrotic, fibro-fatty, calcification and necrotic core, can be identified as they exhibit a defined radiofrequency spectrum, which can be analyzed and mathematically transformed into a color-coded representation of the plaque composition [36].

Therefore, IVUS imaging delivers precise geometric measurements of the coronary wall and lumen and enables the identification of different types of plaques according to their content in lipid, fibrin calcium and necrotic tissues [12,32,37,38]. The evaluation of lipid deposits contents commonly associated to vulnerable plaques and positive remodeling has been used to assess lesion severity [39]. In addition, three-dimensional IVUS image reconstruction is possible and is essential for proper assessment of the longitudinal distribution of the plaque [36], because multiple plaque morphologies varying from a fibrotic stable plaque to sites containing large lipids/necrotic cores can be found in a single arterial segment.

Because of its methodology, IVUS is not subject to the same limitations as angiography. Not only is IVUS more sensitive than angiography for the detection of stenosis, it can also identify diffuse disease and positive remodeling of the vessel wall. Furthermore, since IVUS allows the identification of morphologic characteristics of vulnerable plaques, it may be helpful in the characterization of atherosclerotic plaque formation [31,40] and in the detection of plaques with a high risk of spontaneous rupture [31]. However, coronary angiography is still regarded by many as the principal imaging technique for guiding coronary interventions. Recently, the correlation of coronary artery geometric measurements using both CA and IVUS has been reported [41-43], calling the attention for the value of IVUS alone or in conjugation with VH as precise measurements of plaque geometric parameters and tissue histological characteristics can be obtained with this modality.

2. Methods

2.1. Study design and participants

Individual data and blood samples were obtained from patients enrolled in a prospective study performed at the Cardiology Service of Santa Marta Hospital (CHLC, Lisbon, Portugal). The study was designed to investigate the association of circulating levels of ox-LDL, TNF-α, sFasL and T-lymphocytes with angiographic data and atherosclerotic plaque morphological and biological characteristics.

Patients, men and women aged between 56 and 71 years old with suspected and known coronary artery disease were included in the study. A total of 35 subjects were eligible to participate: 4 patients with ST-elevation myocardial infarction (STEMI), 7 patients with non-ST elevation myocardial infarction (NSTEMI), 11 stable angina (SA) patients, 10 unstable angina (UA) patients and 3 silent ischemia patients (SI). All patients underwent standard diagnostic procedures and treated accordingly. Acute coronary syndrome patients were enrolled in the first 24 hours of hospital admission, although the time period from the onset of chest pain to the intervention was less than 9 hours for the majority of them. Demographic information and history, including traditional risk factors for CAD were obtained at study entry. Evaluations included cardiac testing and imaging, cardiac characteristics and procedures, such as angioplasty and stenting. Coronary angiography and IVUS-VH data was recorded. One pre-specified study lesion was identified in each patient. An anatomical segment containing the entirety of the study lesion was then selected, which could be easily identified based on standard anatomical landmarks on two modalities (CA and IVUS-VH). All patients received standard care therapy after discharge including dual antiplatelet therapy after angioplasty.

Subjects with age above 85, significant co-morbidities as peripheral artery disease or carotid artery disease, known antecedents of malignance or infectious diseases, chronic renal insufficiency, concurrent inflammatory disorders, malignant neoplasm or infection and previous myocardial infarction in the previous 5 years were not enrolled. Also, patients were ineligible if coronary anatomy was inappropriate for IVUS.

The study protocol was approved by the CHLC Ethical Committee board and all patients signed an informed consent accepting their participation before study enrollment.

2.2. Patient characterization

All subjects were characterized demographically, clinically and biochemically (Table I).

Diabetes was diagnosed on the basis of fasting plasma glucose concentration ≥7.0 mmol/l (126 mg/dl) or 2h plasma glucose ≥11.1 mmol/l (200 mg/dl) or confirmed as clinically known and treated diabetes mellitus. Subjects were diagnosed hypertensive if they were documented to have systolic blood pressure ≥140 mmHg and/or diastolic blood pressure ≥90 mmHg or were already on anti-hypertensive therapy. Dyslipidaemia was identified in subjects who had total serum cholesterol level ≥190 mg/dl and/or serum triglycerides ≥180 mg/dl or were on lipid-lowering medication. Smoking was defined as the inhaled use of cigarettes, cigars or pipes in any quantity. Subjects who smoked within the previous year were also defined as smokers.

Patients characterization		
Demographics	Male sex (n, %)	23, 66
	Age (y)	63 (56 – 71)
	Weight (kg)	75 (67 – 80)
	Height (m)	1.7 (1.6 – 1.7)
	BMI (kg/m²)	27.3 (23.7 – 29)
Risk factors / Co-morbidities	Smoking (n, %)	6, 34
	Hypercholesterolemia (n, %)	25, 71
	Arterial hypertension (n, %)	25, 71
	Diabetes mellitus (n, %)	8, 23
Previous medication	Aspirin (n, %)	18, 51
	ACE Inhibitors (n, %)	16, 46
	Anti-platelets (n, %)	14, 40
	β - blockers (n, %)	15, 43
	Statins (n, %)	25, 7
Biochemical analysis	Total cholesterol (mg/dl)	156 (133 – 188)
	LDL (mg/dl)	104 (82 – 127)
	HDL (mg/dl)	36 (27 – 45)
	Triglycerides (mg/dl)	85 (59 – 127)
	Glucose (mg/dl)	111 (95 – 137)
	Leucocytes (x10³/µl)	6.8 (5.4 – 8.5)
	Neutrophils (x10³/µl)	4.4 (3.3 – 5.7)
	Lymphocytes (x10³/µl)	1.8 (1.3 – 2.7)
	Monocytes (x10³/µl)	0.5 (0.3 – 0.8)
	Platelets (x10³/µl)	190 (156 – 235)
	CK (U/l)	84 (47 – 169)
	CRP (mg/l)	5.3 (2.5 – 18.4)
	Pro-BNP (pg/ml)	203 (64 – 916)

Table 1. Patients demographic, clinical and biochemical characterization. Results are presented in median (Q25 – Q75) unless otherwise specified.

2.3. Percutaneous angiography

All patients were clinically evaluated for the extension of coronary artery disease through the characterization of lesion morphology to define the coronary stenosis, the number of diseased vessels, the thrombolysis in myocardial infarction (TIMI) risk score, which refers to the level of coronary blood flow assessed during coronary angiography (ranging from 3 – complete perfusion, to 0 – total occlusion), lesion length and the presence of calcium and/or thrombi in the lesions. The number and type of stents positioned in patients undergoing coronary angiography were also recorded. A coronary stenosis was considered clinically significant (high-grade) as a ≥70% narrowing in the luminal diameter. Multivessel disease was defined when more than one major coronary artery presented high-grade stenosis: left anterior descending artery (LAD); right coronary artery (RCA); left circumflex artery (LCX).

Patients angiographic characterization		
Stenosis (%)		87.5 (70 – 91)
Lesion length (mm)		18.5 (13– 28)
Multivessel (n, %)		6, 19
Diseased vessels (n, %)	0	4, 11
	1	20, 57
	2	7, 20
	3	2, 6
Lesions (n, %)	0	4, 11
	1	17, 49
	2	6, 17
	3	2, 6
	4	4, 11
Culprit vessel (n, %)	LAD / TC	20, 61
	RCA	11, 31
	LCX	2, 6
TIMI score (n, %)	0	1, 3
	3	26, 74
Lesion type (n, %)	A	3, 9
	B	17, 49
	C	2, 6
Lesion morphology (n, %)	Concentric	5, 14
	Eccentric	20, 57

Table 2. Patients angiographic characterization. Results are presented in median (Q25–Q75) unless otherwise specified.

The extent (severity) of CAD was assessed following a graded angiographic system based on previous reports by others [43, 44]. The number of diseased vessels, number of lesions, culprit lesion and TIMI were the contributing parameters. The severity score was calculated on the basis of the sum of individual scores assigned to each parameter assuming normal arteries as grade "0": a) each vessel with ≥70% stenosis lesions contributed as 2, and vessels with <70% stenosis lesions contributed as 1; b) each lesion treated contributed as 1; c) the most severe lesions were graded 3 when occurring in LAD, 2 in RCA and 1 in LCX; d) the TIMI values contributed as 0 = no occlusion to 3 = total occlusion.

2.4. Intravascular ultrasound (IVUS)

The IVUS-VH acquisition was performed using a EagleEye catheter (20 MHz) at pullback speed of 0.5 mm/sec. The IVUS data was recorded for the reconstruction of the radiofrequency backscatter information using In-Vision gold commercial software (Volcano Corporation, USA).

For each lesion, vessel and lumen area data were obtained for every cross-section throughout the region of interest and lesion borders were established using the leading edges of external elastic lamina (EEL) and the luminal contour. Minimal lumen diameter and reference diameter were measured and percentage of diameter stenosis was calculated. The composition of coronary atheroma was assessed using spectral analysis of backscatter RF signals. The percentages of fibrotic, fibro-fatty, calcified and necrotic core were assessed. Atheroma area and volume and were obtained after EEL and lumen diameter (LD) measures were completed at the lumen/plaque boundary and at the media/adventitia boundary in each cross-section forming the region of interest.

Atheroma or plaque area (PA) was determined as the difference between EEL and lumen areas. The plaque burden was calculated as the plaque cross sectional area divided by the EEL area and multiplying by 100. IVUS measurements were recorded at three different regions-of-interest of the selected lesion: larger stenosis region cross-section and distal and proximal cross-sections. Median values and 25% and 75% quartile intervals for the various parameters measured and/or calculated are listed in Table 3.

2.5. Blood sampling and laboratory assays

Peripheral blood was drawn from all patients into blood collection tubes (Vacuette) with appropriate anti-coagulant, and centrifuged at 2500 rpm for 10 minutes. Serum and plasma were collected and stored at -80ºC until analysis, for a period not exceeding 6 months. Samples were thawed only once.

Levels of glucose, creatinine kinase, troponin T, N-terminal pro-brain natriuretic peptide (NT-proBNP) and C-reactive protein (CRP), blood cells count and lipid profile were routinely measured in the hospital. Plasma concentrations of ox-LDL and sFasL and serum concentrations of TNF-α were measured by enzyme-linked immunosorbent assays (ELISA) commercial kits (R&D Systems).

All the assays were performed according to the manufacturer's recommendations. Each sample was measured in duplicate; intra-assay variation among the duplicates for all samples was <10%.

Lymphocyte populations were analyzed by flow cytometry (FASCalibur, BD) in whole blood lysed with lysing solution (BD). The following antibodies were used: PerCP mouse anti-human CD45 (2D1, BD Pharmigen), FITC mouse anti-human CD3 (HIT3a, BD Pharmigen), APC mouse anti-human CD4 (RPA-T4, BD Pharmigen), PE mouse anti-human CD8 (RPA-T8, BD Pharmigen).

Atherosclerotic plaque characterization			
Stenosis (%)		Larger stenosis region	77.6 (65 – 84)
		Proximal region	49 (40 – 58)
		Distal region	48.1 (37 – 59.5)
Fibrotic tissue (%)		Larger stenosis region	58.5 (51 – 75)
		Proximal region	61.7 (48 – 75.5)
		Distal region	59 (43 – 74.5)
Fibro-fatty tissue (%)		Larger stenosis region	9.6 (6.4 – 18)
		Proximal region	13 (5 – 17.5)
		Distal region	9 (4.7 – 20)
Calcified tissue (%)		Larger stenosis region	11 (2.7 – 17)
		Proximal region	6 (0.3 – 14.2)
		Distal region	12.8 (0.5 – 22)
Necrotic core (%)		Larger stenosis region	16.5 (8 – 22)
		Proximal region	17.4 (8 – 24)
		Distal region	16.5 (10 – 24)
Lumen	diameter (mm)	Minimum	2.1 (1.8 – 2.3)
		Maximum	2.4 (2.1 – 3)
		Median	2.2 (1.9 – 2.7)
	area (mm²)		3.8 (2.9 – 5.1)
External elastic lamina	diameter (mm)	Minimum	4.3 (4 – 4.6)
		Maximum	4.9 (4.5 – 5.1)
		Median	4.6 (4.2 – 4.9)
	area (mm²)		17.2 (15 – 19)
Plaque area (mm²)			13 (10 – 15)
Plaque burden (%)			77.4 (65 – 84)

Table 3. Atherosclerotic plaque measurements obtained by IVUS-VH. Results of the plaque morphology and composition are presented in median (Q25 – Q75).

2.6. Statistical analysis

Data were summarized and represented (box-plots) as median and inter-quartiles 25% and 75% (Q25-Q75) for continuous variables and as proportions for categorical variables. Non-continuous variables were analyzed using a 2x2 table and $\chi 2$ test. Continuous variables, such as plaque measures at proximal, distal and larger stenosis region cross-sections of the plaque, transformed into categorical variables based on median values. Differences between classes of variables were compared using a Mann-Whitney test. Associations between variables, angiographic data and IVUS measures were evaluated using non-parametric Spearman correlations.

The calculations were performed using SPSS (v. 19.0, IBM 2010) and linear regressions were made using OriginLab (v. 7.5 SR6, OriginaLab Comp, 2006).

3. Results

The atherosclerotic plaque physical characteristics and composition obtained by IVUS were studied and related with the severity of CAD following CA scores. These parameters were also associated with plaque-related oxidative and inflammation bio-indicators measured in the blood. The inter-relations between the parameters measured are described below.

3.1. Analysis of plaque components along the lesion

The composition of the plaque along its length in terms of fibrotic, fibro-fatty, necrotic and calcified tissues assessed by IVUS-VH can be inferred from data listed in Table 3. Measurements were carried out along the plaque at three plaque regions. Therefore, larger stenosis region, proximal and distal cross-sections were studied.

The variations observed between proximal, distal and larger stenosis region cross-sections did not reach statistical significance, although major variations were also observed in fibro-fatty and calcified tissues. To further analyze the plaque composition, the associations between the fibrotic, fibro-fatty, calcified and necrotic components of the plaque were assessed.

In the overall, high fibrotic and fibro-fatty tissue contents were correlated to low content of calcified tissue and low necrotic core (Fig. 1).

The necrotic core content was positively correlated with calcified tissue (r=0.675, p<0.001). The correlation values were more representative in the region with larger stenosis, although the associations were observed in proximal and distal cross-sections.

Categorizing the plaque necrotic core and calcified tissue contents by the median value, it was confirmed that these two components were significantly associated with the fibrotic and fibro-fatty tissues. Plaques with large areas of necrotic core (≥16.5%) had low percentage of fibrotic (p=0.001) and fibro-fatty (p=0.002) tissues and these levels were significantly different from those in plaques with necrotic core <16.5%. Moreover, the percentage of calcium content increased in plaques with necrotic core content ≥16.5% relative to plaques with necrotic core below 16.5% (p=0.001) (Fig. 2). These differences were valid and equally significant along the plaque length, i.e. for distal, proximal and larger stenosis region cross-sections.

However, when the plaque components were analyzed relative to the calcified tissue content (cut-point and median value of 11%) only the plaque fibrotic content could be discriminated in the larger stenosis region (Q25-Q75=58.8-77.5% fibrotic tissue for calcified tissue <11%; Q25-Q75=33.1-58.7% fibrotic tissue for calcified tissue ≥11%; p<0.001).

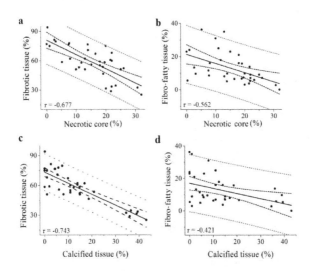

Figure 1. Correlation of necrotic core (a and b) and calcified tissue (c and d) with fibrotic tissue (r=-0.677, p<0.001 and r=-0.743, p<0.001, respectively) and fibro-fatty tissue (r=-0.562, p<0.001, r=-0.421 and p=0.012, respectively) in the larger stenosis region. Solid line represents the linear regression, black dashed lines represent 95% confidence bands and grey dashed lines represent prediction bands.

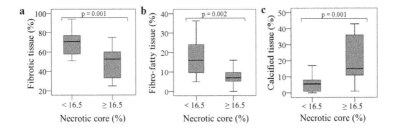

Figure 2. Box-plots of plaque content in fibrotic (a), fibro-fatty (b) and calcified (c) tissues according to the necrotic core levels <16.5% and ≥16.5% in the larger stenosis region.

3.2. Association between plaque components and plaque morphology

Measures of the EEL diameter and area, lumen diameter and area, plaque area and plaque burden were related with the plaque composition in order to assess whether the correlations between these parameters could identify plaque types. It was observed that associations between morphology and components of the plaque varied along the lesion. The relationship between the plaque content in calcified and fibrotic tissues and plaque morphology was only verified in proximal cross-sections of the plaques.

It was observed that the calcified tissue content was positively correlated with the EEL diameter ($r=0.525$, $p=0.001$), the EEL area ($r=0.478$, $p=0.004$) and plaque area ($r=0.442$, $p=0.008$) in proximal cross-sections (see Fig. 3).

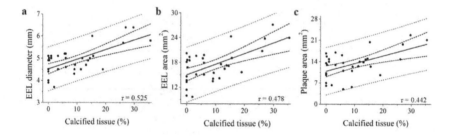

Figure 3. Correlation of calcified tissue content in the proximal region with EEL maximum diameter (a) and plaque area (b). Solid line represents the linear regression, black dashed lines represent 95% confidence bands and grey dashed lines represent prediction bands.

Also in the proximal region of the plaques, the fibrotic content discriminated plaque sizes as expressed by the EEL diameter and area. Both EEL diameter and area were significantly higher for fibrotic tissue percentages below median value (<59%) by report to plaques with fibrotic tissue percentages above median ($p=0.041$) (Fig. 4).

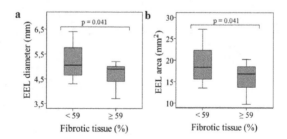

Figure 4. Variations of EEL diameter (a) and area (b) according to fibrotic content <59% and ≥59% in the proximal region.

3.3. Coronary angiography data versus IVUS measures

The IVUS-derived measures of coronary atherosclerotic plaques were evaluated having into account the severity score established with angiographic data. Severity of CAD was found to be unambiguously associated to vessel lumen decrease and increased plaque burden. The severity score was negatively correlated with the plaque geometry IVUS VH-derived measures, such as lumen diameter (r=-0.402, p=0.038) and lumen area (r=-0.419, p=0.03), and positively correlated with plaque burden (r=0.496, p=0.009) as can be depicted in Fig. 5.

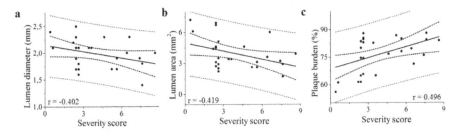

Figure 5. Correlation of angiographic severity with IVUS-derived measures of the atherosclerotic plaque: a) lumen diameter; b) lumen area; and c) plaque burden. Solid line represents the linear regression, black dashed lines represent 95% confidence bands and grey dashed lines represent prediction bands.

3.4. Association of soluble biomarkers and T-cells with IVUS and angiography derived measures

The relationship between the levels of indicators of oxidation and inflammation in the blood circulation with IVUS- and angiography-derived measures of the atherosclerotic plaque was examined with the aim of establishing relevant associations between biomarkers and plaque type.

Indicators of the inflammatory process associated to cell activation and apoptosis, such as TNF-α and sFasL, were determined. Also the concentration of ox-LDL in circulation was assessed as a measure of plaque outflow and inflammation. The variations observed in the concentration levels of these parameters were studied relative to the plaque IVUS-derived measures and angiographic data and severity score.

Several associations were observed between the plaque morphology and components, such as fibrotic, fibro-fatty and necrotic core, with CD4$^+$ and CD8$^+$ T-cell populations and TNF-α, sFasL and ox-LDL concentrations in the blood circulation. Due to the limited number of patients enrolled in this prospective study and to improve statistical results enabling the concurrent evaluation of IVUS and angiographic data, including the severity score, IVUS variables (see variables listed in Table 3) were categorized using the median value as cut-off point.

Following this procedure, and in what concerns soluble biomarkers, it was observed that sFasL, TNF-α and ox-LDL levels in circulation were strongly associated to the median values of lumen and plaque dimensions.

The concentration of TNF-α significantly increased for large plaque areas, as expressed by EEL diameter and area (p=0.05 in both cases), whereas sFasL concentrations increased with diminished lumen diameters (p=0.017), as can be depicted in Fig. 6.

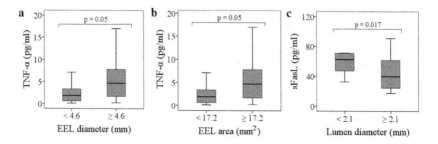

Figure 6. Box-plot representation of the TNF-α and sFasL concentrations relative to indicators of plaque dimensions: a) EEL diameter categories <4.6 mm and ≥4.6 mm; b) EEL area categories <17.2 mm² and ≥17.2mm²; c) Lumen diameter categories <2.1 mm and ≥2.1 mm

The concentrations of ox-LDL in plasma were significantly associated with plaque area as can be depicted in Fig. 7. Large plaque areas, above median value (area ≥13 mm²), were associated with high ox-LDL concentrations whereas plaque areas below 13 mm² were associated with low ox-LDL concentrations, and the differences between median concentration values of ox-LDL in the two groups were significant (p=0.039).

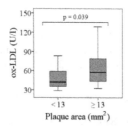

Figure 7. Box-plot representation of ox-LDL concentrations according to plaque area categories <13 mm² and ≥13 mm².

Concerning the plaque components, only the necrotic content assessed in the plaque region with larger stenosis could be associated with TNF-α concentration in circulation. High concentrations of TNF-α were associated with low necrotic core contents contrasting with the significantly lowered TNF-α concentrations (p=0.016) observed in plaques with large necrotic cores (≥16.5%) (Fig. 8)

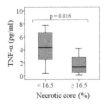

Figure 8. Box-plot representation of TNF-α concentrations according to the necrotic core categories in the larger stenosis region, <16.5 % and ≥16.5 %.

In what concerns T-cell CD3⁺ populations expressing CD4 and CD8, it was observed that the percentage of T-cells expressing CD3CD8 were associated with the plaque dimensions (T-cell CD3⁺CD8⁺ vs EEL diameter r=-0.518, p=0.019; T-cell CD3⁺CD8⁺ vs EEL area r=-0.530, p=0.016). T-cells, both CD3⁺CD4⁺ and CD3⁺CD8⁺, were correlated with the plaque fibrotic and fibro-fatty tissue components along the plaque length, i.e. from distal to proximal regions. Likely, CD3⁺CD4⁺ lymphocytes were positively correlated with fibrotic tissue (r=0.579, p=0.009) whereas CD3⁺CD8⁺ cells were negatively correlated (r=-0.481, p=0.037) (see Fig. 9 a and c).

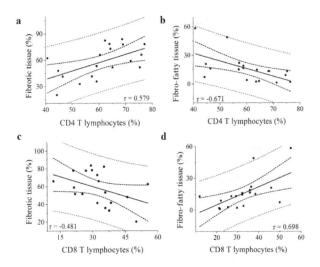

Figure 9. Correlation between plaque fibro-fatty and fibrotic tissue content and CD4⁺ and CD8⁺ T lymphocytes. Solid line represents the linear regression, black dashed lines represent 95% confidence bands and grey dashed lines represent prediction bands.

An opposite relationship was found between fibro-fatty tissue component and CD3$^+$CD4$^+$ lymphocytes (Fig. 9 b and d). The CD3$^+$CD4$^+$ lymphocytes were negatively correlated with fibro-fatty tissue (r =-0.671, p=0.002) and CD3$^+$CD8$^+$ were positively correlated (r=0.698, p=0.001).

4. Discussion

This prospective study showed that plaque composition is related to plaque morphology and these characteristics were associated with the concentration of biomarkers in blood circulation.

Plaques with higher content in necrotic core showed lower fibrotic and fibro-fatty contents and larger areas of calcified tissue. Increased EEL diameter and area were associated to larger fibrotic and calcium contents, linking these two components to plaques protruding in the vessel wall rather than high-stenosis regions. Together these observations suggest that plaque vulnerability is not strictly linked to high-grade stenosis. Also the angiographic disease severity score was associated with plaque burden. This is in agreement with previous studies demonstrating that plaque ruptures typically occur in large and complex plaques [1,30], and that coronary calcification is associated to acute coronary syndromes [37] and independently predicts all-cause mortality in CAD in addition to traditional risk factors [46]. Prior studies reported that shear stress and circumferential wall stress play an important role in plaque rupture [47]. Sano *et al.* [31] demonstrated that the percentage of fibrous area was the most sensitive parameter for classifying the plaques causing acute coronary syndrome. Also the percentage of lipid area was significant in the classification of vulnerable plaques [31]. Evidences are accumulating by coronary angiography and IVUS and other imaging modalities showing that plaque complexity associates to vulnerable plaques [11,31,37]. Therefore, to differentiate vulnerable plaques from stable plaques, the fragile part of the atheromatous plaque is of major interest and both tissue characteristics of coronary plaques and mechanical stresses on coronary plaques should be taken into account.

Plaque rupture is related to the process in which fibrous caps over lipid core become fragile [3]. Several *in vitro* studies support that continuous inflammatory stimulus in the plaque driven by the infiltration of monocytes, macrophages and T-lymphocytes in the lesion, ultimately lead to disintegration of foam cells, and release of cytokines, such as TNF-α, and matrix metalloproteinases [6,7,18-20]. All this causes the destabilization of plaque lipid rich cores and the thinning of the fibrous cap [3,8].

We have preciously demonstrated [48] that the susceptibility of a plaque to rupture is not strictly linked to significant stenosis. This prospective study supports our previous findings as positive associations between plaque dimensions i.e., EEL diameter and area independent of high-stenosis regions, and the concentrations of TNF-α were found. TNF-α is involved in endothelial cells activation and in the inflammatory response amplification [9,20]. Increasing levels of this pro-inflammatory cytokine promote a continuous systemic inflammatory stimulation that can trigger and/or amplify local inflammatory responses and therefore express the extent of vascular inflammation. Also the relationship found between TNF-α concentration in blood and the percentage of necrotic core area suggests an association between an exacerbation of inflammation and the thinning of the fibrous cap with increases of fibrous and fibro-fatty areas as plaque evolves [30,31].

In addition the process of apoptosis is an important mechanism in the pathophysiology of atherosclerosis. Atherosclerotic plaques include large numbers of apoptotic cells and related receptors, such as FasL, which is a type II membrane protein that induces apoptosis when it binds to its membrane receptor Fas. FasL is expressed by activated T lymphocytes, as well as endothelial cells [49]. It was observed in this study that decreases of lumen diameter as occurring in disease exacerbation, favored the elevation of sFasL in circulation. This supports the view that one of the control mechanisms elicited by FasL in CAD may be the prevention of inflammation by destruction of the activated inflammatory cells invading vascular tissues via FasL/Fas-mediated apoptosis [49,50]. In fact, in this study the percentage of T-cells expressing CD4 and CD8 were associated to the percentage of fibrous and fibro-fatty area reinforcing the notion that Th1 cellular immunity is taking place during the disease process [6]. Also, the opposite relationship between the percentage of CD4$^+$ and CD8$^+$ T-cells and the plaque percentage of fibrous and fibro-fatty areas, as observed in this study call the attention for the balanced action of these immune cells in CAD. However, the role of specific immune responses has remained unclear. Evidence is accumulating that T-cells homing the vessel wall contribute to inflammation [6,9] and that T-cell expressing CD4 promote atherosclerosis particularly when activated by LDL modified by oxidative processes [26,27]. The T-cells expressing CD8, when activated, trigger caspase pathways. However, CD4$^+$ and CD8$^+$ T produce different effectors molecules and then effect different cells and pathways, although redundancy of mechanisms has been described pointing to the importance of lymphocyte homeostasis in disease.

The positive association of plaque area with ox-LDL concentrations in plasma can also be considered a marker of plaque instability and/or plaque rupture [51,52] in addition to disease severity. Extensive experimental data shows that ox-LDL is formed in the arterial wall [14,16] contributing to the plaque progression. It is accepted that ox-LDL in circulation is originated in the vessel wall, being their circulating levels strongly associated to angiographically documented CAD [25]. Increases in plaque area, and therefore in regions where lumen decreases relative to circumferential EEL, may favor plaque outflow. In these regions the vessel wall is exposed to shear stress that may contribute to endothelial denuding and plaque cap erosion [47].

The current forms of imaging enable atherosclerosis assessment at the later stage when the vascular morphology has changed dramatically. However, the evaluation of plaque characteristics by angiography and IVUS-VH was associated to circulating biomarkers levels, and these indicators may reflect plaque vulnerability. The *in vivo* identification of plaque vulnerability whether by characterizing its components or by providing measures of oxidative and inflammation markers may improve diagnostic and eventually allow the detection of vulnerable atheroma before rupture. The relations among the plaque components – fibrotic, fibro-fatty calcified and necrotic core – and plaque dimensions, may be important in the characterization of the plaque and in the assessment of its development. Also, circulating ox-LDL, sFasL, TNF-α and lymphocyte populations may be viable targets to follow as they may reflect the global extend of atherosclerosis and may provide useful information on patient's evolution, together with quantitative angiography-derived plaque parameters. The approach may be incorporated in carefully designed clinical studies for the assessment of coronary atherosclerosis.

5. Study limitations

This prospective study is a single-centre study that has a number of limitations. The small number of patients enrolled did not allow association of parameters with clinical presentation. The measurements of biomarkers that entered into the study do not reflect chronic circulating levels, as more than 50% of patients presented with acute coronary syndromes (STEMI, NSTEMI and UA), which transiently alters levels of inflammatory biomarkers. Some of the measurements may be confounded by concomitant treatments (medication, stenting, etc.), which could not be estimated due to the reduced number of patients. We also wish to emphasize that all angiography and IVUS studies are limited to the analysis of a relatively short segment of coronary arterial tree that does not fully reflect disease characteristics elsewhere. The results obtained of plaque components were not confirmed by histology or other diagnostic modalities, such as optical coherent tomography.

6. Conclusions

The present study using angiography and IVUS-VH revealed that the atherosclerotic plaque components and dimensions were related to the concentration of biomarkers in the blood circulation. We reported on the vascular tissue characteristics that may be associated with vulnerable plaques and the incremental value of biomarkers in addition to invasive imaging modalities.

The association of ox-LDL, sFasL and TNF-α circulating levels with lumen dimension and plaque dimension suggest that these indicators may express not only plaque rupture but plaque vulnerability as well. Also the association of TNF-α and T lymphocytes expressing CD4 and CD8 with plaque percentage of fibrous, fibro-fatty, and necrotic core areas may contribute to an in vivo assessment of vascular inflammation and vulnerable plaques and their detection before rupture.

The results suggest that these biomarkers have clinical implications for identifying vulnerable plaques as well as vulnerable patients. Further studies are needed to evaluate the impact of these biomarkers and angiography and IVUS-VH derived measures on clinical presentation.

Acknowledgements

This work was supported by Fundação para a Ciência e Tecnologia (PIC/IC/82734/2007 and SFRM/BPD/6308/2009); and by Liga dos Amigos do Hospital de Santa Marta.

Author details

Catarina Ramos[1], Patrícia Napoleão[2], Rui Cruz Ferreira[3], Cristina Fondinho[3], Mafalda Selas[3], Miguel Mota Carmo[4], Ana Maria Crespo[4] and Teresa Pinheiro[1*]

*Address all correspondence to: murmur@itn.pt

1 IST/ITN Instituto Superior Técnico, Universidade Técnica de Lisboa, Sacavém, Portugal

2 Unidade de Biologia Microvascular e Inflamação, Instituto de Medicina Molecular, Faculdade de Medicina da Universidade de Lisboa, Lisboa, Portugal

3 Serviço Cardiologia, Hospital Santa Marta, Centro Hospitalar Lisboa Central, Lisboa, Portugal

4 Centro de Estudos de Doenças Crónicas, Faculdade de Ciências Médicas, Universidade Nova de Lisboa & Serviço Cardiologia, Hospital Santa Marta Centro Hospitalar Lisboa Central, Lisboa, Portugal

CESAM & Departamento de Biologia Animal, Faculdade de Ciências da Universidade de Lisboa, Lisboa, Portugal

References

[1] Hoffmann U, Moselewski F, Nieman K, Jang IK, Ferencik M, Rahman AM, Cury RC, Abbara S, Joneidi-Jafari H, Achenbach S, Brady TJ, Noninvasive Assessment of Plaque Morphology and Composition in Culprit and Stable Lesions in Acute Coronary Syndrome and Stable Lesions in Stable Angina by Multidetector Computed Tomography, Am Coll Cardiol 2006; 47: 1655– 62

[2] Red-Horse K, Ueno H, Weissman IL, Krasnow MA, Coronary arteries form by developmental reprogramming of venous cells, Nature 2010; 464: 549-553

[3] Stone GW, Maehara A, Mintz GS, The Reality of Vulnerable Plaque Detection, JACC: Cardiovascular Imaging 2011; 4: 902-904

[4] Roger VL, Go AS, Lloyd-Jones DM, Adams RJ,. Berry JD, Brown TM, Carnethon MR, Dai S, de Simone G,. Ford ES, Fox CS, Fullerton HJ, Gillespie C, Greenlund KJ,. Hail-

pern SM, Heit JA, Ho PM, Howard VJ, Kissela BM, Kittner SJ, Lackland DT, Lichtman JH, Lisabeth LD, Makuc DM, Marcus GM, Mozaffarian D, Mussolino ME, Nichol G, Paynter NP, Rosamond WD, Sorlie PD, Stafford RS, Turan TN, Turner MB, Wong ND, Wylie-Rosett J, Heart Disease and Stroke Statistics—2011 Update, Circulation 2011; 123: e18-e209

[5] Ross R, Atherosclerosis — An Inflammatory Disease, N Engl J Med 1999; 340: 115-126

[6] Libby P, Ridker PM, Hansson GK, Inflammation in Atherosclerosis: From Pathophysiology to Practice, J. Am. Coll. Cardiol. 2009; 54: 2129-2138

[7] Galkina E, Ley K, Vascular Adhesion Molecules in Atherosclerosis, Atherosclero Tromb, Vasc Biol 2007; 27: 2292 - 2301

[8] Vancraeynest D, Pasquet A, Roelants V, Gerber BL, Vanoverschelde JJ, Imaging the Vulnerable Plaque, J Am Coll Cardiol 2011; 57: 1961–79

[9] Hansson GK, Inflammation, Atherosclerosis, and Coronary Artery Disease, N Engl J Med 2005; 352: 1685-95

[10] Goldstein JL, Ross MS, Regulation of low-density lipoprotein receptors: implications for pathogenesis and therapy of hypercholesterolemia and atherosclerosis, Circulation 1987; 76: 504-507

[11] Goldstein JA, Demetriou D, Grines CL, Pica M, Shoukfeh M, O'Neill WW, Multiple complex coronary plaques in patients with acute myocardial infarction, New Engl J Med 2000; 343: 915-22

[12] Fayad ZA, Fuster V, Clinical imaging of the high-risk or vulnerable atherosclerotic plaque, Circ. Res. 2001; 89: 305-316

[13] Choi SH, Chae A, Miller E, Messig M, Ntanios F, DeMaria AN, Nissen SE, Witztum JL, Tsimikas S, Relationship Between Biomarkers of Oxidized Low-Density Lipoprotein, Statin Therapy, Quantitative Coronary Angiography, and Atheroma Volume, J Am Coll Cardiol 2008; 52: 24-32

[14] Greco TP, Conti-Kelly AM, Anthony JR, Greco Jr T, Doyle R, Boisen M, Kojima K, Pharm BA, Matsuura E, Lopez LR, Oxidized-LDL/β_2-Glycoprotein I Complexes Are Associated With Disease Severity and Increased Risk for Adverse Outcomes in Patients With Acute Coronary Syndromes, Am J Clin Pathol 2010;133:737-743

[15] Bronas UG, Dengel DR, Influence of Vascular Oxidative Stress and Inflammation on the Development and Progression of Atherosclerosis, Am J of Lifestyle Med 2010; 4: 521 - 534

[16] Tabas I, The Role of Endoplasmic Reticulum Stress in the Progression of Atherosclerosis, Circ Res 2010; 107: 839-850

[17] van Gils JM, Derby MC, Fernandes LR, Ramkhelawon B, Ray TD, Rayner KJ, Parathath S, Distel E, Feig JL, Alvarez-Leite JI, Rayner AJ, McDonald TO, O'Brien KD,

Stuart LM, Fisher EA, Lacy-Hulbert A, Moore KJ, The neuroimmune guidance cue netrin-1 promotes atherosclerosis by inhibiting the emigration of macrophages from plaques, Nature Immunology 2012; 13: 136–143

[18] Mallat Z, Taleb S, Ait-Oufella H, Tedgui A, The role of adaptive T cell immunity in atherosclerosis, J. Lipid Res. 2009; 50: S364–S369

[19] Keaney Jr JF, Immune Modulation of Atherosclerosis, Circulation 2011; 124: e559 - e560

[20] Zernecke A, Weber C, Chemokines in the vascular inflammatory response of athero-sclerosis, Cardiovasc Res 2010; 86: 192 – 201

[21] An G, Wang H, Tang R, Yago T, McDaniel JM, McGee S, Huo Y, Xia L, P-selectin gly-coprotein ligand-1 is highly expressed on Ly-6Chi monocytes and a major determi-nant for Ly-6Chi monocyte recruitment to sites of atherosclerosis in mice, Circulation 2008; 117: 3227–37

[22] Viemann D, Barczyk K, Vogl T, Fischer U, Sunderkötter C, Schulze-Osthoff K, Roth J, MRP8/MRP14 impairs endothelial integrity and induces a caspase-dependent and in-dependent cell death program, Blood 2007; 109: 2453-2460

[23] Ray KK, Morrow DA, Sabatine MS, Shui A, Rifai N, Cannon CP, Braunwald E, Long-Term Prognostic Value of Neopterin: A Novel Marker of Monocyte Activation in Pa-tients With Acute Coronary Syndrome, Circulation 2007; 115: 3071 - 3078

[24] Lopes-Virella MF, Virella G, Clinical Significance of the Humoral Immune Response to Modified LDL, Clin Immunol. 2010; 134(1): 55–65

[25] Tsimikas S, Brilakis ES, Miller ER, McConnell JP, Lennon RJ, Kornman KS, Witztum JL, Berger PB, Oxidized Phospholipids, Lp(a) Lipoprotein, and Coronary Artery Dis-ease, N Engl J Med 2005; 353: 46-57.

[26] Greco TP, Conti-Kelly AM, Greco Jr T, Doyle R, Matsuura E, Anthony JR, Lopez LR, Newer Antiphospholipid Antibodies Predict Adverse Outcomes in Patients With Acute Coronary Syndrome, Am J Clin Pathol 2009; 132: 613-620

[27] Ludewig B, Freigang S, Jäggi M, Kurrer MO, Pei YC, Vlk L, Odermatt B, Zinkernagel RM, Hengartner H, Linking immune-mediated arterial inflammation and cholester-ol-induced atherosclerosis in a transgenic mouse model, Proc Natl Acad Sci U S A 2000; 97: 12752–7

[28] Peters RJ, Kok WE, Pasterkamp G, Von Birgelen C, Prins M, Serruys PW, Videoden-sitometric quantitative angiography after coronary balloon angioplasty, compared to edge-detection quantitative angiography and intracoronary ultrasound imaging, Eur Heart J 2000; 21: 654–661

[29] Leber AW, Knez A, von Ziegler F, Becker A, Nikolaou K, Paul S, Wintersperger B, Reiser M, Becker CR, Steinbeck G, Boekstegers P, Quantification of Obstructive and

Nonobstructive Coronary Lesions by 64-Slice Computed Tomography, J Am Coll Cardiol 2005; 46; 147-154

[30] Böse D, von Birgelen C, Erbel R, Intravascular Ultrasound for the Evaluation of Therapies Targeting Coronary Atherosclerosis, J Am Coll Cardiol 2007; 49:925–32

[31] Sano K, Kawasaki M, Ishihara Y, Okubo M, Tsuchiya K, Nishigaki K, Zhou X, Minatoguchi S, Fujita H, Fujiwara H, Assessment of Vulnerable Plaques Causing Acute Coronary Syndrome Using Integrated Backscatter Intravascular Ultrasound, J Am Coll Cardiol 2006; 47: 734–41

[32] Springer I, Dewey M, Comparison of multislice computed tomography with intravascular ultrasound for detection and characterization of coronary artery plaques: a systematic review, Eur J Radiol 2009; 71: 275-82.

[33] Gao D, Ning N, Guo Y, Ning W, Niu X, Yang J, Computed tomography for detecting coronary artery plaques: a meta-analysis, Atherosclerosis 2011; 219: 603-9.

[34] van der Giessen AG, Toepker MH, Donelly PM, Bamberg F, Schlett CL, Raffle C, Irlbeck T, Lee H, van Walsum T, Maurovich-Horvat P, Gijsen FJ, Wentzel JJ, Hoffmann U, Reproducibility, accuracy, and predictors of accuracy for the detection of coronary atherosclerotic plaque composition by computed tomography: an ex vivo comparison to intravascular ultrasound, Invest Radiol. 2010; 45: 693-701

[35] Rodriguez-Granillo GA, García-García HM, Mc Fadden EP, Valgimigli M, Aoki J, de Feyter P, Serruys PW. In Vivo Intravascular Ultrasound-Derived Thin-Cap Fibroatheroma Detection Using Ultrasound Radiofrequency Data Analysis. J Am Coll Cardiol 2005; 46: 2038–42

[36] Calvert PA, Obaid DR, O'Sullivan M, Shapiro LM, McNab D, Densem CG, Schofield PM, Braganza D, Clarke SC, Ray KK, West NEJ, Bennett MR, Association Between IVUS Findings and Adverse Outcomes in Patients With Coronary Artery Disease, JACC: Cardiovascular Imaging, 2011; 4: 894-901

[37] Nakamura T, Kubo N, Funayama H, Sugawara Y, Ako J, Momomura S, Plaque characteristics of the coronary segment proximal to the culprit lesion in stable and unstable patients, Clin. Cardiol. 2009; 32: e9–e12

[38] Stähr PM, Höfflinghaus T, Voigtländer T, Courtney BK, Victor A, Otto M, Yock PG, Brennecke R, Fitzgerald PJ, Discrimination of Early/Intermediate and Advanced/Complicated Coronary Plaque Types by Radiofrequency Intravascular Ultrasound Analysis, Am J Cardiol. 2002; 9: 19-23

[39] Costa MA, Kozuma K, Gaster AL, van Der Giessen WJ, Sabate M, Foley DP, Kay I, Ligthart J, Thayssen P, van den Brand MJ, de Feyter PJ, Serruys P, Three dimensional intravascular ultrasonic assessment of the local mechanism of restenosis after balloon angioplasty. Heart 2001; 85: 73–79.

[40] Amato M, Montorsi P, Ravani A, Oldani E, Galli S, Ravagnani PM, Tremoli E, Baldassarre D, Carotid intima-media thickness by B-mode ultrasound as surrogate of

coronary atherosclerosis: correlation with quantitative coronary angiography and coronary intravascular ultrasound findings, European Heart Journal, 2007; 28: 2094–2101

[41] Voros S, Rinehart S, Qian Z, Vazquez G, Anderson H, Murrieta L, Wilmer C, Carlson H, Taylor K, Ballard W, Karmpaliotis D, Kalynych A, Brown C, Prospective Validation of Standardized, 3-Dimensional, Quantitative Coronary Computed Tomographic Plaque Measurements Using Radiofrequency Backscatter Intravascular Ultrasound as Reference Standard in Intermediate Coronary Arterial Lesions, J Am Coll Cardiol Intv 2011; 4: 198–208

[42] Peters RJG, Kok WEM, Pasterkamp G, von Birgelen C, Prins M, Serruys PW on behalf of the PICTURE study group. Videodensitometric quantitative angiography after coronary balloon angioplasty, compared to edge-detection quantitative angiography and intracoronary ultrasound imaging. Eur Heart J 2000; 21: 654–661

[43] Leber AW, Knez A, von Ziegler F, Becker A, Nikolaou K, Paul S, Wintersperger B, Reiser M, Becker CR, Steinbeck G, Boekstegers P, Quantification of Obstructive and Nonobstructive Coronary Lesions by 64-Slice Computed Tomography A Comparative Study With Quantitative Coronary Angiography and Intravascular Ultrasound. J Am Coll Cardiol 2005; 46: 147–54.

[44] Naruko T, Furukawa A, Yunoki K, Komatsu R, Nakagawa N, Matsumura Y, Shirai N, Sugioka K, Takagi M, Hozumi T, Itoh A, Haze K, Yoshiyama M, Becker AE, Ueda M. Increased expression and plasma levels of myeloperoxidase are closely related to the presence of angiographically-detected complex lesion morphology in unstable angina. Heart 2010; 96: 1716-1722.

[45] Yun KH, Mintz GS, Farhat N, Marso SP, Taglieri N, Verheye S, Foster MC, Margolis MP, Templin B, Xu K, Dressler O, Mehran R, Stone GW, Maehara A, Relation Between Angiographic Lesion Severity, Vulnerable Plaque Morphology and Future Adverse Cardiac Events (from the Providing Regional Observations to Study Predictors of Events in the Coronary Tree Study), Am J Cardiol. 2012; 110: 471-7.

[46] Budoff MJ, Shaw LJ, Liu ST, Weinstein SR, Mosler TP, Tseng PH, Flores FR, Callister TQ, Raggi P, Berman DS. Long-term prognosis associated with coronary calcification. J Am Coll Cardiol 2007;49:1860-70.

[47] Cheng GC, Loree HM, Kamm RD, Fishbein MC, Lee RT. Distribution of circumferential stress in ruptured and stable atherosclerotic lesions: a structural analysis with histopathological correlation. Circulation 1993;87: 1179 – 87.

[48] P. Napoleão, M. Selas, C. Ramos, A. Turkman, V. Andreozzi, M. Mota Carmo, A. M. Viegas-Crespo, R. Cruz Ferreira, T. Pinheiro. The Role of Inflammatory Biomarkers in the Assessment of Coronary Artery Disease. In: Branislav Baskot (ed.) Coronary Angiography - Advances in Noninvasive Imaging Approach for Evaluation of Coronary Artery Disease: InTech; 2011. p281-314.

[49] Sata M, Walsh K. TNF-alpha regulation of Fas ligand expression on the vascular en-
      dothelium modulates leukocyte extravasation. Nat Med 1998; 4 :415-420.

[50] Blanco-Colio LM, Martín-Ventura JL, Tuñón J, García-Camarero T, Berrazueta JR,
      Egido J. Soluble Fas ligand plasma levels are associated with forearm reactive hyper-
      emia in subjects with coronary artery disease: a novel biomarker of endothelial func-
      tion? Atherosclerosis. 2008;201:407-12.

[51] P. Napoleão, M. Selas, A. Toste, A. Turkman, V. Andreozzi, A.M. Viegas-Crespo, T.
      Pinheiro, R. Cruz Ferreira. Serial changes of oxidized low-density lipoprotein associ-
      ated with culprit vessel in ST-elevation myocardial infarction – a promising marker?
      Rev Port Cardiol 2009;28:303-308.

[52] M. Mota Carmo, P. Napoleão, S. Andrade, A.M. Selas, C. Freixo, A Turkman, V. An-
      dreozzi, A.M. Viegas-Crespo, T. Pinheiro, R.C. Ferreira, High Oxidized LDL Asso-
      ciate to Low T-Lymphocytes in Acute Myocardial Infarction. Circulation 2010;122:
      E161.

Chapter 2

Reduced Consumption of Olive Oil: A Risk for Ischemic Heart Disease?

Massimo Cocchi and Giovanni Lercker

Additional information is available at the end of the chapter

1. Introduction

Comparing the nutritional content of food to individual health status, there are several considerations that can be informative and raise troubling concerns. For many decades, researchers have investigated the relationships between health status and consumption of extra virgin olive oil. Extra virgin olive oil (and oleic acid) is considered important for the prevention and coronary heart disease. While the biomolecular aspects involving G protein need further research, oleic acid levels in platelets may be a discriminating factor, together with linoleic and arachidonic acid, for coronary heart disease. There is still a huge debate regarding the effects of oleic acid alone or in combination with antioxidants.

Coronary Heart Disease (CHD) is the main cause of death and morbidity in industrialized countries. The incidence of myocardial infarction, however, is highly variable, with lower rates in Mediterranean countries compared to those in northern Europe, USA, or Australia [1]. Paradoxically, the low incidence of myocardial infarction occurs in spite of a high prevalence of classical cardiovascular risk factors [2].

Olive oil is the primary source of fat in the Mediterranean diet. The beneficial effects of olive oil on CHD have now been recognized, and are often attributed to the high levels of monounsaturated fatty acids (MUFA) [3]. Indeed, in November 2004, the US Federal Drug Administration (FDA) allowed a claim on olive oil labels concerning "the benefits on the risk of coronary heart disease of eating about two tablespoons (23 g) of olive oil daily, due to the MUFA in olive oil" [4].

2. A crucial element for a healthy heart: oleic acid and platelets

Oleic acid, and especially that obtained from pressing olives, is a crucial element in the prevention of ischemic cardiovascular disease, as has been demonstrated by a series of international scientific activity. Fatty acids other than n-3 Polyunsaturated Fatty Acids (PUFAs) can interact with the metabolism of eicosanoids and potentially influence platelet function. For example, there is evidence that diets rich in unsaturated fatty acids, such as linoleic acid and oleic acid, can also decrease thromboembolic risk by replacing arachidonic acid in platelet phospholipids, decreasing, at least in vitro, the production of thromboxane A_2 [TXA2] and platelet aggregation. However, there is little conclusive evidence that platelet function in vivo is affected by diet [5].

Oleic acid has been found to be a potent inhibitor of platelet aggregating factor (PAF) and serotonin secretion. Consequently, in order to understand the molecular mechanisms of oleic acid action, the effects of this fatty acid on several biochemical events associated with platelet aggregation induced by PAF have been investigated. In particular, it has been found that oleic acid causes a decrease in the levels of phosphatidyl inositide phosphate (PIP) and PIP2, which is associated with an inhibition of platelet aggregation induced by PAF. These results suggest that inhibition of the PAF response by oleic acid may be at least one of the steps involved in signal transduction [6].

Several literature reports have further suggested that olive oil may inhibit platelet function. This possible effect is of interest for two reasons. First, it may contribute to the apparent anti-atherogenic effects of olive oil, and second, it may invalidate the use of olive oil as an inert placebo in studies of platelet function. After exposure to olive oil, platelet aggregation and TXA2 release decreased, and the content of platelet membrane oleic acid increased significantly; platelet membrane arachidonic acid content was found to significantly decrease. This suggests that excess of oleic acid impairs the incorporation of arachidonic acid into platelet phospholipids.

Olive oil also has an inhibitory effect on various aspects of platelet function, which might be associated with decreased risk for heart disease, although fish intake also plays a protective role [7].

The beneficial effects of olive oil can be attributed to its high content of oleic acid (70-80%). The consumption of olive oil increases the levels of oleic acid in cell membranes, which helps to regulate the structure of membrane lipids through the control of signal-mediated G-protein, causing a reduction in blood pressure [8].

In rats, cardiovascular tissues treated with 2-OHOA (hydroxy oleic acid) show activation of cAMP in response to activation of Gsα protein, which can be attributed to increased expression of Gsα proteins. As a result, there is significant reduction in systolic blood pressure [9]. The involvement of Gs alpha protein is also of interest considering the hypothesis forwarded by Cocchi, Tonello, Rasenick and Hameroff in psychiatric disorders as depression, suicide etc. (private meeting, 2008). In light of the below model, the role of Gsα protein in ischemic heart disease merits further investigation.

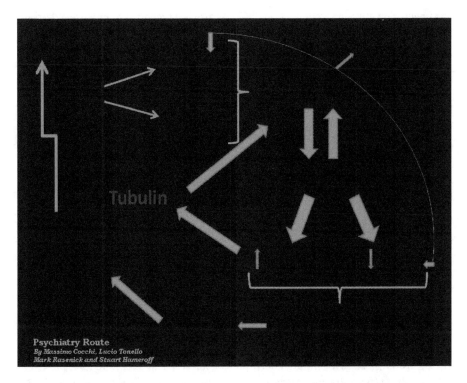

Figure 1. Description of selected biochemical and biomolecular events potentially involved in psychiatric disorders.

In figure 1, the molecular depression hypothesis described by Cocchi et al. [10], Donati et al. [11] and Hameroff and Penrose [12] is shown. Because of the possible similarity of the platelet to neurons, membrane viscosity can modify Gsα protein status. The Gsα protein is associated with tubulin. Depending on local membrane lipid composition, tubulin may serve as a positive or negative regulator of phosphatidylinositol bisphosphate hydrolysis (PIP2) similar to G proteins. Tubulin is known to form high-affinity complexes with certain G proteins. The formation of these complexes allows tubulin to activate Gsα protein and creates a system whereby elements of the cytoskeleton can influence G-protein signaling. Rapid changes in membrane lipid composition or the cytoskeleton can modify neuronal signaling through such a mechanism.

Protein kinase C (PKC) activation (Figure 2) is preceded by a number of steps, originating from the binding of an extracellular ligand that activates a G-protein on the cytosolic side of the plasma membrane. This G-protein, using guanosine triphosphate (GTP) as an energy source, then activates protein kinase C (PKC) via the phosphatidylinositol bisphosphate (PIP2) intermediate, which is shown as the diacylglycerol DAG/IP3 complex. Several studies have shown that a reduced functionality of the serotonin (5-HT) transporter in some psychiatric disorders, such as obsessive-compulsive disorder (OCD), may be related to alterations in its regulation at an intracellular level. PKC has also been reported to provoke a decrease in the number of 5-HT transporter proteins. The increased activity of PKC in OCD may be the result of increased activity of the phosphatidylinositol pathway.

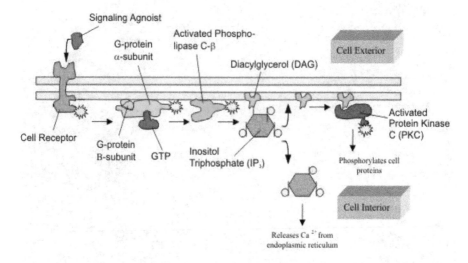

Figure 2. Description of PKC activation. Adapted from Alberts et al. [13].

The exclusive use of olive oil during food preparation seems to offer significant protection against ischemic heart disease, in spite of poor clinical conditions, lifestyle and other characteristics of individuals [14]. In addition, several historical papers have reported on the positive effects of olive oil on CHD.

In 1985, Mattson and Grundy [15] reported that olive oil reduces HDL cholesterol, which plays a protective, anti-atherogenic function, favoring the elimination of LDL-cholesterol. In 1986, Sirtori et al. [16] have shown that in addition to its effects on cholesterol and atherosclerosis, olive oil has preventive action on thrombosis and platelet aggregation. High intake of olive oil is not harmful, and reduces the levels of LDL-cholesterol, but not HDL [17 - 25].

3. Oleic acid and Atherogenesis

Atherosclerosis is considered to be an inflammatory disease [26], and endothelial dysfunction occurs early in the development of the pathology. Traditional risk factors for atherosclerosis promote endothelium activation, which induces adhesion and trans-endothelial migration of monocytes [26]. Several inflammatory mediators are released by the endothelium such as the eicosanoids derived from n-6 PUFA arachidonic acid. These include prostaglandin E2 (PGE2), leukotriene B4, a chemoattractant and neutrophile activator, thromboxane, a potent vasoconstrictor, and platelet-aggregating factor [27].

Monocytes and macrophages are critical cells present in all stages of atherosclerosis. In addition to promoting LDL oxidation through free radical production, they also secrete proinflammatory cytokines such as IL-1 and Tumor Necrosis Factor (TNF), which stimulate the expression of adhesion molecules such as intercellular cell adhesion molecule-1 (ICAM-1), vascular-cell adhesion molecule-1 (VCAM-1), and E-selectin [25]. Circulating monocytes are attracted by these molecules and adhere to the endothelium, from which they transmigrate to the subendothelial space. Once within the endothelium, monocytes differentiate into macrophages, which in turn scavenge oxidized LDL, thus becoming foam cells and lead to plaque formation.

The proinflammatory response releases a principal messenger from macrophages, namely cytokine IL6. After engagement of its receptor on the liver, IL6 promotes the secretion of C Reactive Protein (CRP), a prototypic marker of inflammation [28, 29]. Serum IL6 and CRP have been shown to be predictive of CHD. Altered levels of serum CRP, IL6, and ICAM-1 have been associated with progression of atherosclerosis, and IL6 has been shown to be a good predictor of progressive peripheral atherosclerosis [30, 31].

The inflammatory protection of diets rich in oleic acid has been attributed to a decrease in the content of LDL linoleic acid [32]. The low susceptibility of oleic acid to oxidation, and the scavenging capacity of minor compounds in olive oil, can decrease the activation of proinflammatory transcription factors, such as nuclear factor-kappa B (NFkB), through a reduction of reactive oxygen spices and peroxyl radicals [33]. In this regard, it has been reported that consumption of meals enriched in olive oil do not activate NFkB in monocytes in contrast to meals rich in butter and walnut-enriched meals [34]. Studies on oleic acid enriched liposomes and vascular endothelium exposed to oleic acid, however, suggest a protective mechanism of oleic acid on free radical generation, oxidative damage to lipids, and inflammatory activity [35, 36].

Recent data suggest that oleic acid is not the only agent responsible for the anti-inflammatory properties of olive oil. In experimental studies, minor components of the unsaponifiable fraction of olive oil, such as alfa-tocopherol, beta-sitosterol, and triterpenes, in addition to phenolic compounds, have all been shown to have both anti-inflammatory and anti-endothelial activation properties [37]. The results of a meta-analysis of 14 studies carried out during 1983–1994 showed that the replacement of SFA by oils enriched in MUFA or PUFA had similar effects on total, LDL, and HDL cholesterol, whereas PUFA-enriched oil had a slight triglyceride-lowering effect [38]. Dubois et al. [39] showed that increasing the amount of fat up to 50 g led to stepwise increases in the postprandial rise of serum triglycerides, while the ingestion of 15 g fat had no effect on postprandial lipemia or lipoproteins in healthy adults. A meal containing 31 g of fat induced considerably less variations in lipemia, chylomicrons, and lipoproteins than a 42 g fat meal [39]. A single dose of 25 mL olive oil was not found to promote postprandial lipemia [40], in contrast to 40 mL and 50 mL doses [41, 42] with no effect on the phenolic content of the olive oil.

Abia et al. [43] reported that virgin olive oil intake resulted in lower postprandial triacylglyceride-rich-lipoprotein (TRL) levels and a faster disappearance of TRL-TG from blood, compared to intake of sunflower oil with a high content of oleic acid. Chylomicrons produced after olive oil [44, 45] or n-3 PUFA [46] ingestion seem to enter the circulation more rapidly, and cleared at a faster rate, in comparison to those produced after intake of fats rich in SFA or PUFA. Although fat intake appears to be the major nutritional determinant of the postprandial triglyceride response, it is also influenced by other dietary components, including fiber, glucose, starch, and alcohol in a meal [47].

The oxidative modification of LDL plays a key role in development of atherosclerosis and CHD. Oxidation of lipids and lipoproteins present in LDL leads to a change in the lipoprotein conformation by which LDL are more facilitated to enter the monocyte/macrophage system of the arterial wall, and promote the atherosclerotic process [48]. It is currently believed that oxidized LDL are more damaging to the arterial wall than native LDL [49]. Elevated concentrations of circulating oxidized LDL show a positive relationship with the severity of acute coronary events [50, 51]. They are also independently associated with carotid intima-media thickness [52] and are predictors for CHD both in CHD patients [53] and the general population [54]. Several studies have been performed comparing the effects of MUFA-rich diets on the susceptibility of LDL to oxidation with those of PUFA- or carbohydrate-rich diets. Oleate-rich LDL have been shown to be less susceptible to oxidation than linoleate rich LDL [55-61].

4. Depression and Ischemic Heart Disease: a common role for oleic acid?

Because of the particular role of platelets on depressive and thrombogenetic risk, our group has investigated the platelet fatty acid profile in three groups of subjects: healthy (n=60), ischemic (n= 50) and depressive (n= 84). The aim of the study was to understand which fatty acid could be utilized as markers of ischemic cardiovascular pathology and depressive disorder, and to classify subjects using an artificial neural network (ANN). All the ANNs tested gave essentially the same result. However, one type of ANN, known as Self-Organizing Map (SOM), [62, 63, 64], gave additional information by allowing the results to be described in a two-dimensional plane with potentially informative border areas. The central property of the SOM is that it forms a nonlinear projection of a high-dimensional data manifold on a regular, low-dimensional (usually 2D) grid.

A series of repeated and independent SOM simulations, with the input parameters being changed each time, led to the finding that the best discriminating map was that obtained by inclusion of the following three fatty acids: palmitic acid (C16:0), linoleic acid (C18:2 *n*-6) and arachidonic acid (C20:4 *n*-6) for depressive subjects and oleic acid (C18:1), linoleic acid and arachidonic acid for ischemic subjects [10, 65-67] (Figures 3, 4).

5. A case study

A 42-year-old female with a very high familial risk for ischemic cardiovascular disease (one sister 34 years old died of heart attack; another sister, 48 years old, heart attack; uncle, two infarctions; mother, 69 years old, died of heart attack; aunt, 59 years old, died of heart attack), was submitted to a classic complete functional cardiovascular investigation which resulted negative. The subject is a heavy smoker, cholesterol: 230 mg/dl, HDL: 84 mg/dl. Framingham score: 13 (low risk score). Platelet levels of oleic acid, linoleic acid and arachidonic acid were analyzed using the SOM designed for ischemic patients, and the concentrations of those fatty acids were entered in the SOM. The subject detailed information on the study and provided informed consent. The patient's fatty acid triplet, tested in the SOM, gave the following result (Figure 5).

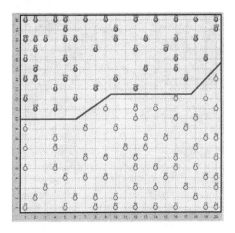

Figure 3. SOM classification of depressive subjects (red) against normal subjects (green). Platelet arachidonic acid $(C_{20:4})$, palmitic acid $(C_{16:0})$, and linoleic acid $(C_{18:2})$ can discriminate depression and have diagnostic power.

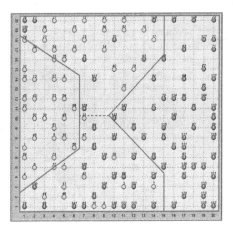

Figure 4. SOM classification of ischemic subjects (red) against normal subjects (green). Platelet oleic acid $(C_{18:1})$, arachidonic acid $(C_{20:4})$, linoleic acid $(C_{18:2})$ can discriminate ischemia and have diagnostic power.

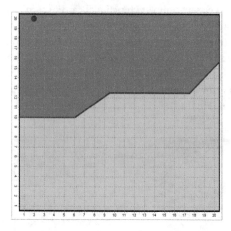

Figure 5. Position of the patient according to the three fatty acids (oleic, linoleic and arachidonic) on the SOM, which classifies ischemic patients.

This result was compared with the SOM classification of normal and pathologic subjects, as shown in figure 4. The patient was asked to submit herself to a Coronary TAC and the images showed "Interventricular Anterior (IVA) branch: small mixed plaque in the proximal tract, 33% of the lumen" (radiological diagnosis). The result suggests the opportunity to select young high risk subjects to evaluate not only the diagnostic power of the SOM, but also the possibility for early diagnosis of plaque formation. A large trial is necessary to validate this result, but based on the classical rules of Evidence Based Medicine, it is very difficult to obtain approval from an ethic's committee.

Medical science has not yet fully understood or accepted the use of the ANN mathematic models in relation to experimental conditions, which are still strongly linked to traditional protocols. The task of finding biomarkers according to the rules dictated by Evidence Based Medicine requires the elimination of selection bias, and leads to selection of a population that may be clinically unrealistic. The characteristics of the above-described method nonetheless allow the analysis to be carried out, and permit to find differences among subsets of the population.

The first fundamental consequence of the use of fatty acids is that an extremely effective and practical diagnostic tool can be obtained, with a strong tolerance to "noise". Secondly, the choice of specific fatty acids and their relative strength in the classification by the SOM allows investigating more in-depth investigation of the problem and helps in understanding the disease from the biochemical point of view.

6. Commonalities between CHD and depression

To demonstrate the powerful grouping capacity of the SOM, we created a new network where all three groups were inserted and grouped simultaneously on the basis of the characteristics of the triplets previously highlighted, which were all different from one another [68] (Figure 6).

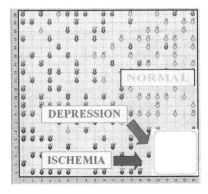

Figure 6. Simultaneous classification, using the SOM, of three groups of subjects (normal, depressive and ischemic). In the right corner of the map, ischemic and depressive subjects are mixed and have, in common, a low level of platelet oleic acid.

As shown by the SOM, it is possible that reduced amounts of oleic acid not only are critical in the biochemical classification of ischemic heart disease, but are also common to a condition that characterizes a relationship between depression and ischemia [69]. It seems possible that levels of C18:1 in platelets dominate in ischemia, and are linked to depression. Furthermore, it can be conjectured that there are two different types of depression, namely classical and ischemia-induced according to the findings of different platelet membrane viscosity and its effect at the biomolecular level. [10-12, 70]. The relationships between depression and ischemic heart disease have been widely studied [71, 72]. Interestingly, Weyers and Colquhoun [73] reported improvements in depressive symptoms in patients with CHD after consumption of olive oil.

7. Do we eat enough extra virgin olive oil?

The question then arises as to whether there is sufficient consumption of olive oil and oleic acid in the Italian population. Knowing that oleic acid can significantly change the composition of platelet fatty acids, which are crucial in the genesis of plaque formation, and can significantly alter the amount of oleic acid in platelet membranes, an experiment on a large group of pigs (80 Duroc x Large White) was performed [74]. Four groups of pigs were studied, 20 animals each, which received four diets containing different lipid fractions, as follows:

Diet 1: corn oil (low linoleic acid.), diet 2: corn oil (medium linoleic acid.), diet 3: sunflower oil (high oleic acid.), diet 4: sunflower oil (high oleic acid) + palm oil (high palmitic acid). The diets fed to animals, to meet the needs for growth, had the following lipid composition (Table 1):

Period (kg)	Diet	EE	C16:0	C18:0	C18:1n9	C18:2n6	C18:3n3
50 - 90	1	2.70	13.13	2.05	31.07	50.90	2.59
50 - 90	2	2.86	14.37	2.04	26.40	54.54	2.42
50 - 90	3	5.30	8.91	2.39	56.47	30.23	1.27
50 - 90	4	5.37	18.67	8.36	39.99	30.86	1.40
90 - 120	1	2.63	12.83	1.72	31.60	51.15	2.38
90 - 120	2	2.57	14.16	1.94	25.76	54.96	2.55
90 - 120	3	5.56	8.81	2.44	57.12	29.73	1.26
90 - 120	4	5.62	20.02	9.26	39.41	29.59	1.12
120 - 160	1	2.83	13.32	1.69	30.46	52.00	2.41
120 - 160	2	2.89	13.75	1.88	25.65	56.29	2.35
120 - 160	3	5.74	8.54	2.10	57.18	30.91	1.07
120 - 160	4	5.76	19.71	9.25	39.16	30.25	1.17

Table 1. Ether extract (% dry Matter) and fatty acid composition of lipid fractions

Fatty Acids		C16:0	C18:0	C18:1n9	C18:2n6	C18:3n3	C20:4
Diet 1	Media s.d.	28.51[a]	32.00	17.38 [B]	9.30	0.63a	12.19 [AB]
		1.84	10.70	5.63	3.40	0.36	5.18
Diet 2	Media s.d.	27.73 [ab]	29.01	18.0 [B]	9.07	0.48ab	15.6 [A]
		1.47	8.48	3.17	2.88	0.29	4.52
Diet 3	Media s.d.	27.00[ab]	27.78	24.93 [A]	9.37	0.34[b]	10.59[B]
		2.07	8.12	6.78	3.10	0.25	4.48
Diet 4	Media s.d.	26.51[b]	32.04	19.36 [B]	9.32	0.51[ab]	12.25[AB]
		2.63	11.07	5.43	3.64	0.32	4.27
P		<0.05	n.s.	<0.01	n.s.	<0.05	<0.01

Table 2. Mean values ± SD of platelet fatty acids in the different treatment groups

The platelet fatty acids (Table 2) were plotted as for ischemic and normal human subjects in the SOM for ischemia (Figure 7).

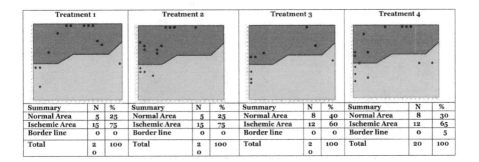

Treatment 1			Treatment 2			Treatment 3			Treatment 4		
Summary	N	%	Summary	N	%	Summary	N	%	Summary	N	%
Normal Area	5	25	Normal Area	5	25	Normal Area	8	40	Normal Area	8	30
Ischemic Area	15	75	Ischemic Area	15	75	Ischemic Area	12	60	Ischemic Area	12	65
Border line	0	0	Border line	0	0	Border line	0	0	Border line	0	5
Total	20	100	Total	20	100	Total	20	100	Total	20	100

Figure 7. By increasing the oleic acid content in diets is possible to move pig platelets, in agreement with the fatty acid triplet [66, 67], from the pathologic (red area) to the normal (green area) area.

It is feasible to obtain similar results in humans. If one considers the characteristics descri-bed for the pig model of atherosclerosis [75], and applying similar characteristics to humans, it can be assumed that we should consume a quantity of oleic acid, and consequently, extra virgin olive oil, that is at least twice that of current levels. To demonstrate this, we made simple considerations based on the purchase of olive oil in Italy (Data provided by the Isti-tuto di Servizi per il Mercato Agricolo Alimentare (ISMEA).

Based on data provided and taking into account that the value derived from the table should be increased by 40%, since about 40% of purchase data were excluded, the consump-tion of extra virgin olive oil for each Italian is on average, about 11.76 grams of oleic acid daily, considering that olive oil is on average value about 70% oleic acid. This value is even likely to be less, as much oil is also used for frying, and therefore cannot be included as part of raw consumption. While this quantity is very small, there are also regional differences be-tween the north and south of Italy.

This observation is also related to the observation that current eating behavior does not al-low large consumption of olive oil. It should be remembered that meals eaten out of the household, often consisting of a sandwich, make it difficult to consume extra virgin olive oil in larger quantities. While the eating habits of rural areas may still be able to compensate this situation, there is an increasing trend to gradually move away from such traditions.

Recently, we investigated the consumption of olive oil in a restaurant in the Center-North of Italy, (2750 subjects in one month). The average consumption of olive oil was 1.8 g per cus-tomer per month, which corresponds to about 1.26 g of oleic acid. Together with the above cited data, this results confirms that olive oil is not consumed in large quantities. Given this, as Ancel Keys pointed out, one wonders if the Mediterranean diet is still a model of health, considering the consumption of extra virgin olive oil.

Systematic name	Trivial name	Shorthand designation	Molecular weight	Melting point (°C)
butanoic	butyric	4:0	88.1	-7.9
pentanoic	valeric	5:0	102,1	-19
hexanoic	caproic	6:0	116.1	-3.4
octanoic	caprylic	8:0	144.2	16.7
nonanoic	pelargonic	9:0	158.2	12.5
decanoic	capric	10:0	172.3	31.6
dodecanoic	lauric	12:0	200.3	44.2
tetradecanoic	myristic	14:0	228.4	53.9
hexadecanoic	palmitic	16:0	256.4	63.1
heptadecanoic	margaric (daturic)	17:0	270.4	61.3
octadecanoic	stearic	18:0	284.4	69.6
eicosanoic	arachidic	20:0	312.5	75.3
docosanoic	behenic	22:0	340.5	79.9
tetracosanoic	lignoceric	24:0	368.6	84.2
cis-9-hexadecenoic	palmitoleic	16:1(n-7)	254.4	0.5
cis-9-octadecenoic	oleic	18:1(n-9)	282.4	16.2
trans-9-octadecenoic	elaidic	tr18:1(n-9)	282.4	43.7
cis-11-octadecenoic	cis-vaccenic (asclepic)	18:1(n-7)	282.4	39
cis-9-eicosenoic	gadoleic	20:1(n-11)	310.5	25
cis-13-docosenoic	erucic	22:1(n-9)	338.6	33.4
9,12-octadecadienoic	linoleic	18:2(n-6)	280.4	-5
6,9,12-octadecatrienoic	γ-linolenic	18:3(n-6)	278.4	
9,12,15-octadecatrienoic	α-linolenic	18:3(n-3)	278.4	-11
8,11,14-eiosatrienoic	dihomo-γ-linolenic	20:3(n-6)	306.5	
5,8,11,14-eicosatetraenoic	arachidonic	20:4(n-6)	304.	-50
6,912,15-octadecatetraenoic	stearidonic	18:4(n-3)	276.4	-57
5,8,11,14,17-eicosapentaenoic	EPA	20:5(n-3)	302.5	-54
7,10,13,16,19-docosapentaenoi	DPA	22:5(n-3)	330.6	
4,7,10,13,16,19-docosahexaenoic	DHA	22:6(n-3)	328.6	-44

(see: http://216.239.59.104/search?q=cache:qTHq_xfePkIJ:www.cyberlipid.org/fa/acid0001.htm+Aitzetm
%C3%BCller+K&hl=it)

Table 3. Selected chemical and physical characteristics of fatty acids

8. Chemical and technological considerations about oleic acid

Fatty acids have different functions in living organisms, including the structural one, which are determined by the length of their hydrocarbon chain and the presence or absence of double bonds. Hydrocarbon chain length, in the same conditions of unsaturation, is directly proportional to the melting point (as well as the boiling point) (Table 3). The solubility in water (Table 4) and unsaturation, for the same chain length, is inversely proportional to the melting point (see Table 3), with very few exceptions.

Carbon number	Solubility
2	Infinite
4	Infinite
6	9.7
8	0.7
10	0.15
12	0.055
14	0.02
16	0.007
18	0.003

Table 4. Fatty acid solubility in water at 20°C (in grams per liter)

These chemical differences are determined in large part by chemical and physical interactions that exist when molecules are close enough to unsaturate them. In the case of fatty acids, the possibility to join molecules depends only on the hydrocarbon chain (Van der Waals forces), which is facilitated when it is saturated and more difficult when unsaturated (especially at the point of unsaturation). The longer and more linear the chain, the greater the interaction, and the more unsaturated it will be, consequently, the interaction will be lower. When fatty acids are part of a triglyceride or phospholipid, the effect occurs in a similar manner and therefore, in biological membranes, a greater or lesser chance of interaction corresponds to greater or lesser "fluidity" of the membrane, which is proportional to more or less functionality (permeability).

At room temperature, in terms of membrane structure, fatty acids are important, and the ones that are more widespread in nature are those with 18 total carbon atoms, especially unsaturated. Modulation of proper membrane fluidity requires that some fatty acids are relatively "rigid", such as palmitic and stearic acid, with a preference for the former since it has a lower melting point and thus is more effective in bringing about small changes.

One of the most important aspects of biological systems that protect themselves through membranes is the preservation of integrity of the membrane itself, which is subject to contact with chemical reactive oxygen species (ROS), and capable of chemically attacking the unsaturated zone of the molecule. Greater effectiveness is related to a greater level of unsaturation, leading to subsequent breakage of the molecule with increased membrane fragility. For these reasons, the membrane is associated with a series of antioxidants, whose action is linked to their position in the membrane [75]. Oleic acid is the least oxidizable among unsaturated fatty acids (Table 5), and is also not too fluid or too rigid, and is thus suitable for prolonging membrane stability [76, 77].

FATTY ACID	1) AUTOXIDATION	2) AUTOXIDATION	PHOTOSENSITIZED OXIDATION (PHOTOXIDATION)
SATURATED	1	1	
MONOENES	10	100	1.1 (32,000)*
DIENES	100	1200	2.9 (1600)*
TRIENES	200	2500	3.5
TETRAENES**	300		
PENTAENES**	400		
HESAENES**	500		

* In brackets ratio between photoxidation and autoxidation is shown

** Hypothesis based on physical-chemical behavior

Table 5. Oxidation rate of several unsaturated fatty acids [Modified from Gunstone et al. [76]]

The rate of oxidation between various unsaturated fatty acids shown in Table 5 appears increased between oleic acid (monoenes) and linoleic acid (dienes), but upon increasing the unsaturation (trienes), the variation is much less pronounced. In biological systems, the position of the fatty acid in glycerides or phospholipids [77] appears to influence the rate of oxidation, and is slower when inserted in position 2, or in the β position of the molecule. In the case of olive oil, as in all vegetable fats (Table 6), the 2 position is occupied by unsaturated fatty acids, and is more available in that position because it can directly cross the intestinal wall of the 2-monoglycerides, resulting from digestion of glycerides by pancreatic lipase. In particular, on a molar basis, 83% of unsaturated fatty acids, in position 2 of triglycerides in olive oil, is occupied by oleic acid.

For extra virgin olive oil, its total unsaturation makes it particularly stable (Table 7) [79, 80] so that appropriate conservation, which is further prolonged by the presence of numerous and effective natural antioxidants (biophenol), is still present after refining, in contrast to other oils.

Fat or Oil source	Fatty acid position	14:0	16:0	18:0	18:1	18:2	18:3	20:0	22:0
Women milk*	1	3.2	16.1	15.0	46.1	11	0.4		
	2	7.3	58.2	3.3	12.7	7.3	0.6		
	3	7.1	6.2	2.0	49.7	2.0	1.6		
Women milk	1	18.2	20.0	73.9	42.5	33.3	15.4		
	2	41.5	72.3	16.3	11.7	22.1	23.1		
	3	40.3	7.7	9.9	45.8	44.5	61.5		
Cow milk	1	11	36	15	21	1			
	2	20	33	6	14	3			
	3	7	10	4	15	<1			
Pig	1	1	10	30	51	6			
	2	4	72	2	13	3			
	3		7		73	8			
Cow	1	4	41	17	20	4	1		
	2	9	17	9	41	5	1		
	3	1	22	24	37	5	1		
Cocoa butter	1		34	50	12	1			
	2		2	2	87	9			
	3		37	53	9				
Groundnut	1		14	5	59	18		1	-
	2		1	<1	58	39		-	-
	3		11	5	57	10		4	6
Corn	1		18	3	27	50	1		
	2		2	<1	26	70	<1		
	3		13	3	31	51	1		
Soya	1		14	6	23	48	9		
	2		1	1	21	70	7		
	3		13	6	28	45	8		
Olive	1		13	3	72	10	<1		
	2		1	-	83	14	1		
	3		7	4	74	5	1		

Mol % = molar percentage

*Relative GC area % (http://www.cyberlipid.org/index.htm); ** Sørensen A.D.M. et al., 2010 [78]

Table 6. Main fatty acid (mol %) distribution in the three positions of glycerine molecule of the corresponding triacylglycerols (triglycerides) of several fats and oils.

Fattyacids	Caprylic (C8:0)	Capric (C10:0)	Lauric (C12:0)	Mirystic (C14:0)	Palmitic (C16:0)	Stearic (C18:0)	Oleic (C18:1)	Linoleic (C18:2)	Linolenic (C18:3)	Eicosenoic (C20:1)	Total Unsaturation[a] (unstability factor)	Iodine number
Oil from:												
Groundnut				ND-0.1	8.0-14.0	1.0-4.5	35.0-69.0	12.0-43.0	0-0.3	0.7-1.7	200-481	86-107
Rapeseed (0 erucic)				ND-0.2	2.5-7.0	0.8-3.0	51.0-70.0	15.0-30.0	5.0-14.0	0.1-4.3	320-630	105-126
Safflower				ND-0.2	5.3-8.0	1.9-2.9	8.4-21.3	67.8-83.2	ND-0.1	0.1-0.3	700-740	136-148
Safflower (HO)				ND-0.2	3.6-6.0	1.5-2.4	70.0-83.7	9.0-19.9	ND-0.2	0.1-0.5	175-270	80-100
Sunflower		ND-0.1		ND-0.2	5.0-7.6	2.7-6.5	14.0-39.4	48.3-74.0	0-0.3	0-0.3	531-766	118-141
Sunflower (HO)				ND-0.1	2.6-5.0	2.9-6.2	70.0-90.7	2.1-20.0	ND-3.0	0.1-0.5	118-270	78-90
Corn		ND-0.3		ND-0.3	8.6-14.0	ND-3.3	20.0-42.0	34.0-65.6	0-1.2	0.2-0.6	400-481	103-135
Olive (CODEX)					7.5-20.0		55.0-83.0	3.5-21.0	Max 1.0	Max 0.4	163-285	75-94
Soya Bean		ND-0.1		ND-0.2	8.0-13.5	2.5-5.4	17.0-30.0	48.0-59.0	4.5-11.0	0-0.5	600-840	124-139
Grape seed				ND-0.3	5.5-11.0	3.0-6.5	12.0-28.0	58.0-78.0	0-1.0	0-0.3	596-802	128-150
Fat from:												
Cocoa butter					22.6-30.4	30.2-36.0	29.2-36.4	1.3-4.0	ND-0.5		370-380	34-40
Coconut	4.6-10	5.0-8.0	45.1-53.2	16.8-21.0	7.5-10.2	2.0-4.0	5.0-10.0	1.0-2.5	ND-0.2	ND-0.2	24-34	6.3-10.6
Palm			ND-0.5	0.5-2.0	39.3-47.5	3.5-6.0	36.3-44.0	9.0-12.0	ND-0.5	ND-0.4	130-391	50.0-55.0
Palm olein			0.1-0.5	0.5-1.5	38.0-43.5	3.5-5.0	39.8-46.0	10.0-13.5	ND-0.6	ND-04	158-187	56
Palm stearin			0.1-0.5	1.0-2.0	48.0-74.0	3.9-6.0	15.5-36.0	3.0-10.0	ND-0.5	ND-0.4	76-270	33
Palm kernel	2.4-6.2	2.6-5.0	45.0-55.0	14.0-18.0	6.5-10.0	1.0-3.0	12.0-19.0	1.0-3.5	ND-0.2	ND-0.2	33-51	14.1-21.0

[a] Total unsaturation is calculated as the relative percentage of single fatty acid for a different factor, for each unsatura-tion, the degree is proportional to the oxidative instability. The factors utilized were: 1 for monounsaturated, 10 for diunsaturated and 20 for triunsaturated fatty acids. HO =high oleic. ND = not detectable

Table 7. Main fatty acid composition of fats and oils

Not all olive oils have the same concentration of oleic acid. The International Olive Oil Council (IOOC) has dictated that the content of oleic acid in olive oils can vary from 55% to 83% of total fatty acids [81]. The regulations of the European Community do not indicate the amount of oleic acid in olive oil, but simply indicate the specifications of several other pa-rameters that are useful for detecting fraud and require the distinction between various commercial products obtained from olive processing.

Among these, extra virgin oils are those that must have the highest quality. Extra virgin olive oils with the highest content of oleic acid have always been regarded as those with the highest quality, but only because of their higher stability during storage, as a consequence of the low reactivity of oleic acid compared with polyunsaturated fats. The Food and Drug Administration (FDA) has stated (November 1, 2004) that U.S. consumption of 23 g of olive oil each day (about two tablespoons) helps in prevention of cardiovascular diseases [4].

Today, there are other sources of oil high in oleic acid, such as safflower, sunflower and canola (the new name for rapeseed oil low in erucic acid), and therefore based solely on the content of oleic acid, these sources would also be optimal in this regard. However, the reputation of olive oil as a healthy product is most likely due to the presence of the numerous "minor elements" contained within [82, 83]. Among these minor components, several compounds are worthy of mention including biophenols, which consists of phenols and polyphenols with high antioxidant and antiradical activity, some triterpene alcohols, phytosterols, squalene, and tocopherols. These latter are considered important because of the content of vitamin E, and for their ability to facilitate the assimilation of polyunsaturated fatty acids: 1 mg allows the assimilation of 1 g of polyunsaturated fatty acids [84].

The discovery of health effects from the minor components in olive oil has led to a large gap in the nutritional properties of edible oils. In fact, oils from seeds, subject to refining, loose many minor components and do not have the health properties that the corresponding matrix has. The technology for olive processing influences the quality and organoleptic characteristics of the final product, which is not always considered by industrial operators as much of the scientific knowledge is particularly new. The olive oil is encapsulated in small drops (10-30 micrometers) within vacuoles with a polysaccharide wall: oil droplets, during processing, are released in crushing and come into contact with the other components of olives during grinding of the paste. It is the prolonged contact with the oil-pasta that allows joining of small droplets such that they can then leave the dough during the separation process that emulsifies all the minor components in oil.

Therefore, time and temperature of processing can also affect the final product, and even if the starting characteristics of the olives are similar they can yield very different products. Moreover, during the same oil-paste stage, enzyme activities are capable of forming the fragrance of the oil through a series of biochemical steps that, in part, may reduce the antioxidant ability of biophenol components and their effects on health. Therefore, choices made during the processing of olives should take these effects into consideration.

There are several hundred olive cultivars grown in Italy, which can produce many oils that have a very different composition, although all can be considered of excellent quality. In particular, the richness in antioxidants (especially biophenols) can affect characteristics of the oil in terms of taste, storage stability, and health properties. Even if much scientific knowledge has been learned about olive production and processing technology, there are still many questions that must be answered in order to improve the quality, especially those related to health, of the oils obtained by processing olives

9. Conclusion

The ability to transform, by the action of delta9-desaturase, stearic acid to oleic acid, and vice versa makes oleic acid very useful for the modulation of the fluidity (and functionality)

of cell membranes. Recalling that the fatty acid composition of platelets can be correlated with depression and also with ischemia [85], we can consider the oil obtained from olive processing such as the lipid substrate better balanced with respect to the fatty acid unsaturations, for the platelet membrane composition of normal individuals.

We must remember that the presence of high concentrations of oleic acid from olive oil is one of the stabilizing factors against oxidative modification, in both cases, for the oil itself and for cell membranes. Furthermore, the oil from olives when is classified as extra virgin, possesses a wealth of biophenols, powerful antioxidants predominantly of antiradical type, which further increase the stability of the oil and, more or less directly, even of the membrane lipids.

Olive oil, and, particularly an extra virgin olive oil-rich diet, decreases prothrombotic activity, and modify platelet adhesion, coagulation, and fibrinolysis. The wide range of antiatherogenic effects associated with olive oil consumption can help to justify the low rate of cardiovascular mortality found in southern European Mediterranean countries, in comparison with other western countries, despite a high prevalence of CHD risk factors. Experimental evidence confirms a critical role of reduced levels of oleic acid in platelets in ischemic subjects with a diagnostic discriminant capacity from normal subjects [85]. At present, although traditional cardiovascular risk factors are under revision, a new field of research in platelets, and in particular oleic acid and its relationship with linoleic and arachidonic acid, should be pursued. The mechanisms by which olive oil exerts its beneficial effects merit further investigation, and additional studies are required to document the benefits of olive oil consumption on primary endpoints for cardiovascular disease. In this regard, consumption of extra virgin olive oil and daily intake of oleic acid should, however, be promoted.

Author details

Massimo Cocchi[1,2] and Giovanni Lercker[3]

1 "Paolo Sotgiu" Institute for research in Quantitative & Quantum Psychiatry & Cardiology, L.U.de.S University, Lugano, Switzerland

2 Department of Medical Veterinary Sciences, University of Bologna, Italy

3 DISA, University of Bologna, Italy

References

[1] Tunstall-Pedoe, H. Kuulasmaa, K. Mahonen, M. Tolonen, H. Ruokokoski, E. Amouyel, P. Contribution of trends in survival and coronary-event rates to changes in coronary heart disease mortality: 10-year results from 37 WHO MONICA project

populations. Monitoring trends and determinants in cardiovascular disease. Lancet, 1999, 353: 1547–57.

[2]   Masia, R. Pena, A Marrugat, J. Sala, J. Vila, J. Pavesi, Covas, M. Aubo, Elosua, C. R. High prevalence of cardiovascular risk factors in Gerona, Spain, a province with low myocardial infarction incidence. REGICOR Investigators. J Epidemiol Community Health, 1998, 52: 707–15.

[3]   Covas, MI. Olive oil and the cardiovascular system. Pharmacological Research, 2007, 55: 175–186.

[4]   US Food and Drug Administration. Press Release P04-100. November 1, 2004. http://www.fda.gov/bbs/topics/news/2004/NEW01129.htlm. Accessed on October 28, 2006.

[5]   Kris-Etherton, P M.; Mustad V. Derr J.A. Effects of dietary stearic acid on plasma lipids and thrombosis, Nutrition Today. 1993, 28: 30-38.

[6]   Nunez, J Randon, C Gandhi, A Siafaka-Kapadai, MS Olson and DJ Hanahan: The inhibition of platelet-activating factor-induced platelet activation by oleic acid is associated with a decrease in polyphosphoinositide metabolism, Journal of Biological Chemisty, Volume 265, n° 30, October 25, pp18330-18338, 1990.

[7]   Barradas, M.A. Christofides, J.A. Jeremy, J.Y. Mikhailidis, D.P. Fry, D.E. Dandona, P. The Effect of Olive Oil Supplementation on Human Platelet Function, Serum Cholesterol-Related Variables and Plasma Fibrinogen Concentrations: A Pilot Study, Nutrition Research, 1990, 10: 403-411.

[8]   Teres, S. Barcelo-Coblijn, G. Benet, M. Alvarez, R. A, Bressani, R. Halver, J. E. Escriba, P. V. Oleic acid content is responsible for the reduction in blood pressure induced by olive oil. PNAS. 2008, 105: 13811-13816.

[9]   Alemany R. Terés S., Baamonde C., Benet M., Vögler O., Escribá P. V. 2-Hydroxyoleic Acid. A New Hypotensive Molecule, Hypertension. 2004, 43: 249-54.

[10] Cocchi, M., Tonello, L. Tsaluchidu, S. Puri, B.K. The use of artificial neural networks to study fatty acids in neuropsychiatric disorders. BMC Psychiatry. 2008, 8(Suppl. 1):S3. doi: 10.1186/1471-244X-8-S1-S3.

[11] Donati, R.J. Dwivedi, Y. Roberts, R.C. Conley, R.R. Pandey, G.N. Rasenick, M.M. Postmortem Brain Tissue of Depressed Suicides Reveals Increased Gs Localization in Lipid Raft Domains Where It Is Less Likely to Activate Adenylyl Cyclase. J. Neurosci. 2008, 28:3042-3050.

[12] Hameroff, S.R. Penrose, R. Orchestrated reduction of quantum coherence in brain microtubules: A model for consciousness. In: SR Hameroff, A Kaszniak and AC Scott (eds.) Toward a Science of Consciousness - The First Tucson Discussions and Debates. MIT Press, Cambridge, UK. 1996, 507-540.

[13] Hameroff, S.R. The "conscious pilot"-dendritic synchrony moves through the brain to mediate consciousness. J. Biol. Phys. 2009, Published online: doi: 10.1007/s10867-009-9148-x.

[14] Alberts B., Bray D., Lewis J., Raff M., Roberts K., Watson JD. Molecular Biology of the cell. Garland Publishing, 1994.

[15] Mattson, F.H. Grundy, S. M. Comparison of effects of dietary saturated, monounsaturated, and polyunsaturated fatty acids on plasma lipids and lipoproteins in man. J Lipid Res. 1985, 26:194-202.

[16] Sirtori, C. R. Tremoli, E. Gatti, E. Montanari, G. Sirtori, M. Colli, S. Gianfranceschi, G. Maderna, P. Dentone, C. Z. Testolin, G. Galli, C. (). Controlled evaluation of fat intake in the Mediterranean diet: comparative activities of olive oil and corn oil on plasma lipids and platelets in high-risk patients. Am. J. Clin. Nutr. 1986, 44: 635-642.

[17] Carmena, R. Ascaso, J.F. Camejo, G. Varela, G. Hurt-Camejo, E. Ordovas, J.M. Martinez-Valls, J. Bergström, M. Wallin, B. Effect of olive oil and sunflower oils on low density lipoprotein level, composition, size, oxidation and interaction with arterial proteoglycans. Atherosclerosis, 1996, 125: 243-255.

[18] Mata, P. Alvarez-Sala, L. A. Rubio, M. J. Nun O. J. De Oya, M. Effects of long-term monounsaturated- vs polyunsaturated-enriched diets on lipoproteins in healthy men and women. Am. J. Clin. Nutr. 1992, 55: 846–850.

[19] Nicolaïew, N. Lemort, N. Adorni, L. Berra, B. Montorfano, G. Rapelli, S. Cortesi, N. Jacotot, B. Comparison between Extra Virgin Olive Oil and Oleic Acid Rich Sunflower Oil: Effects on Postprandial Lipemia and LDL Susceptibility to Oxidation. Ann. Nutr. Metab. 1998, 42: 251-260.

[20] Mensink, R. De Groot, M. Vanden Broeke, L. Severigen-Nobels, A. Demacker, P. Katan, M. Effect of monounsaturated fatty acids vs. complex carbohydrates on serum lipoproteins and apolipoproteins in healthy men and women. Metabolism. 1989, 38: 172-178.

[21] Carmena, R. Ros, E. Gómez Gerique, J. A. Masana, L. Ascaso, J. F. Betancort, P. Ecomen daciones para la prevención de la arteriosclerosis en España. Documento Oficial de la Sociedad Española de Arteriosclerosis (Recommendations for atherosclerosis prevention in Spain). In: Official document by The Spanish Atherosclerosis Society Clin Invest Arterios clerosis 1, 1989, 1–9.

[22] Grundy, S. M. Comparison of monounsaturated fatty acids and carbohydrates. N Eng J Med. 1986, 314: 745-748.

[23] Grundy, S. M. Flosentin, L. Nix, D. Whelan, M. F. Comparison of monounsaturated fatty acids and carbohydrates for reducing raised levels of plasma cholesterol in man. Am J Clin Nutr. 1988, 47: 965-969.

[24] Mattson, F.H. Grundy, S.M. Comparison of effects of dietary saturated, monounsaturated, and polyunsaturated fatty acids on plasma lipids and lipoproteins in man J Lipid Res. 1985, 26: 194-202.

[25] Keys, A. Coronary heart diseases in seven countries. Circulation, 1970, 41 sppl 1: 163–211.

[26] Ross, R. Atherosclerosis: an inflammatory disease. N Eng J Med. 1999, 340: 115–26.

[27] Dogne, J.M. de Leval, X. Hanson, J. Frederich, M. Lambermont, B. Ghuysen, A. Casini, A. Masereel, B. Ruan, K. H., Pirotte, B. Kolh, P. New developments on thromboxane and prostacyclin modulators. Part I. Thromboxane modulators. Curr Med Chem. 2004, 11: 1223–41.

[28] Jialal, I. Devaraj, S. Venugopal, S.K. C-reactive protein: risk marker or mediator in atherothrombosis? Hypertension, 2004, 44: 6–11.

[29] Jialal, I. Devaraj, S. Inflammation and atherosclerosis: the value of the high sensitivity C-reactive protein assay as a risk marker. Am J Clin Pathol. 2001, 116(Sup):S108–15.

[30] Kritchevsky, S.B. Cesari, M. Pahor, M. Inflammatory markers and cardiovascular health in older adults. Cardiovasc Res. 2005, 66: 265–75.

[31] Tzoulaki, I. Murray G.D., Lee, A.J. Rumley, A. Lowe, G.D. Fowkes, F.G. C-reactive protein, interleukin-6, and soluble adhesion molecules as predictors of progressive peripheral atherosclerosis in the general population: Edinburgh Artery Study. Circulation 2005, 112: 976–83.

[32] Tsimikas, S. Philis-Tsimikas, A. Alexopoulos, S. Sigari, F. Lee, C. Reaven, P.D. LDL isolated from Greek subjects on a typical diet or from American subjects on an oleate-supplemented diet induces less monocyte chemotaxis and adhesion when exposed to oxidative stress. Arterioscler Thromb.Vasc Biol. 1999, 19: 122–30.

[33] Thanos, D. Maniatis, T. NFkB: a lesson in family values. Cell, 1995, 80: 529–32.

[34] Bellido, C. Lopez-Miranda, J. Blanco-Colio, L.M. Pérez-Martínez, P. Muriana F.J. Martín-Ventura, J.L. Marín, C. Gomez, P. Fuentes, F. Egido, J. Pérez-Jiménez, F. Butter and walnuts, but not olive oil, elicit postprandial activation of nuclear transcription factor kappaB in peripheral blood mononuclear cells. Am J Clin Nutr. 2004, 80: 1487–91.

[35] Lee, C. Barnett, J. Reaven, P.D. Liposomes enriched in oleic acid are less susceptible to oxidation and have less proinflammatory activity when exposed to oxidizing conditions. J Lipid Res. 1998, 39: 1239–47.

[36] Massaro, M. basta, G. Lazzerini, G. Carluccio, M. A. Bosetti, F. Solaini, G. Visioli, F. Paolicchi, A. De Caterina, R. Quenching of intracellular ROS generation as a mechanism for oleate-induced reduction of endothelial activation and early atherogenesis. Thromb Haemost. 2002, 88: 335–44.

[37] Perona, J.S. Cabello-Moruno, R. Ruiz-Gutierrez, V. The role of virgin olive oil compo-
      nents in the modulation of endotelial function. J Nutr Biochem, 2006, 17: 429–45.

[38] Gardner, C.D. Kraemer, H.C. Monounsaturated versus polyunsaturated dietary fat
      and serum lipids. A meta-analysis. Arterioscler Thromb Vasc Biol. 1995, 15: 1917–27.

[39] Dubois, C. Armand, M. Azais-Braesco, V. Portugal, H. Pauli, A.M. Bernard, P.M.
      Latge, C. Lafont, H. Borel, P. Lairon, D. Effects of moderate amounts of emulsified
      dietary fat on postprandial lipemia and lipoproteins in normolipidemic adults. Am J
      Clin Nutr. 1994, 60: 374–82.

[40] Weinbrenner, T. Fitò, M. Farre-Albaladejo, M. Saez, G. Rijken, P. Tormos, C. Coolen,
      S. de la Torre, R. Covas M.I. Bioavailability of phenolic compounds from olive oil
      and oxidative/ antioxidant status at postprandial state in healthy humans. Drugs Exp
      Clin Res. 2004, 30: 207–14.

[41] Fitò, M. Gimeno, E. Covas M.I. Mirò, E. Lòpez-Sabater, M.C. Farrè, M. de la Torre,
      Jmarrugat, R. Postprandial and short-term dietary intervention effects of virgin olive
      oil ingestion on the oxidative/antioxidative status. Lipids 2002, 37: 245–51.

[42] Covas, M.I. de la Torre, K. Farrè-Albaladejo, M. Kaikkonen, J. Fitò, M. Lopez-Sabater,
      C. Pujadas-Bastardes, M.A. Joglar, J. Weinbrenner, T. Lamuela-Raventós, R.M., de la
      Torre, R. Postprandial LDL phenolic content and LDL oxidation is modulated by
      olive oil phenolic compound in humans. Free Rad Biol Med. 2006, 40: 608–16.

[43] Abia, R. Pacheco, Y.M. Perona, J.S. Montero, E. Muriana, F.J. Ruiz-Gutierrez, V. The
      metabolic availability of dietary triacylglycerols from two high oleic oils during the
      postprandial period does not depend on the amount of oleic acid ingested by healthy
      men. J Nutr. 2001, 131: 59–65.

[44] Roche, H.M. Zampelas, A. Knapper, J.M. Webb, D. Brooks, C. Jackson, K.G. Wright,
      J. W. Gould, B. J. Kafatos, A. Gibney, M.J. Williams, C.M. Effect of long-term olive oil
      dietary intervention on postprandial triacylglycerol and factor VII metabolism. Am J
      Clin Nutr 1998, 68: 552– 60.

[45] Williams, C.M. Dietary interventions affecting chylomicron and chylomicron rem-
      nant clearance. Atherosclerosis 1998, 141(Suppl 1):S87–92.

[46] Rivellese, A.A. Iovine, C. Ciano, O. Costagliola, L. Galasso, R. Riccardi, G. Vaccaro,
      O. Nutrient determinants of postprandial triglyceride response in a population-
      based sample of type II diabetic patients. Eur J Clin Nutr. 2006, 60: 1168–73.

[47] Witztum, J.L. Steinberg, D. Role of oxidized low density lipoprotein in atherogenesis.
      J Clin Invest. 1991, 88: 1785–92.

[48] Navab, M. Berliner, J.A. Watson, A.D. Hama, S.Y. Territo, M.C. Lusis, A.J. Shih, D.M.
      Van Lenten, B.J. Frank, J.S. Demer, L.L. Edwards, P.A. Fogelman, A.M. The Ying and
      Tang of oxidation in the development of the fatty streak. Arterioscler Thromb Vasc
      Biol. 1996, 16: 831–42.

[49] Holvoet, P. Mertens, A. Verhamme, P. Bogaerts, K. Beyens, G. Verhaeghe, R. Collen, D. Muls, E. Van de Werf, F. Circulating oxidized LDL is a useful marker for identifying patients with coronary artery disease. Arterioscler Thromb Vasc Biol. 2001, 21: 844–8.

[50] Weinbrenner, T. Cladellas, M. Covas, M.I. Fitò, M. Tomas, M. Senti, M. Bruguera, J. Marrugat, J. High oxidative stress in patients with stable coronary heart disease. Atherosclerosis, 2003, 168: 99–106.

[51] Liu, M.L. Ylitalo, K. Salonen, R. Salonen, J.T. Taskinen, M.R. Circulating oxidized low-density lipoprotein and its association with carotid intima-media thickness in asymptomatic members of familial combined hyperlipidemia families. Arterioscler ThrombVasc Biol. 2004, 24: 1492–7.

[52] Toshima, S. Hasegawa, A. Kurabayashi, M. Itabe, H. Takano, T. Sugano, J. Shimamura, K. Kimura, Michishita, J.I. Suzuki, T. Nagai, R. Circulating oxidized low density lipoprotein levels. A biochemical risk marker for coronary heart disease. Arterioscler Thromb Vasc Biol 2000, 20: 2243–7.

[53] Meisinger, C. Baumert, J. Khuseyinova, N. Loewel, H. Koenig, W. Plasma oxidized low-density lipoprotein, a strong predictor for acute coronary heart disease events un apparently healthy, middle-aged men from the general population. Circulation, 2005, 112: 651–7.

[54] Parthasarathy, S. Khoo, J.C. Miller, E. Barnett, J. Witztum, J.L. Steinberg, D. Low density lipoprotein rich in oleic acid is protected against oxidative modification: implications for dietary prevention of atherosclerosis. Proc Natl Acad Sci USA. 1990, 87: 3894–8.

[55] Berry, E.M. Eisenberg, S. Harats, D. Friedlander, Y. Norman, Y. Kaufmann, N.A. Norman, Y. Stein, Y. Effects of diets rich in monounsaturated fatty acids on plasma lipoproteins – the Jerusalem Nutrition Study: high MUFAs vs high PUFAs. Am J Clin Nutr.1991, 53: 899–907.

[56] Reaven, P. Parthasarathy, S. Grasse, B.J. Miller, E. Steinberg, D. Witztum, J.L. Effects of oleate-rich and linoleate-rich diets on the susceptibility of low density lipoprotein to oxidative modification in mildly hypercholesterolemic subjects. J Clin Invest. 1993, 91: 668–76.

[57] Bonanome, A. Pagnan, A. Biffanti, S. Opportuno, A. Sorgato, F. Dorella, M. Maiorino, M. Ursini, F. Effect of dietary monounsaturated and polyunsaturated fatty acids on the susceptibility of plasma low density lipoproteins to oxidativemodification. Arterioscler Thromb. 1992, 12: 529–33.

[58] Abbey, M. Belling, G.B. Noakes, M. Hirata, F. Nestel, P.J. Oxidation of lowdensity lipoproteins: intraindividual variability and the effect of dietary linoleate supplementation. Am J Clin Nutr. 1993, 57: 391–8.

[59] Baroni, S.S. Amelio, M. Sangiorgi, Z. Gaddi, A. Battino, M. Solid monounsaturated diet lowers LDL unsaturation trait and oxidisability in hypercholesterolemic (type IIb) patients. Free Radic Res. 1999, 30: 275–85.

[60] Mata, P. Varela, O. Alonso, R. Lahoz, C. de Oya, M. Badimon, L. Monounsaturated and polyunsaturated n-6 fatty acid-enriched diets modify LDL oxidation and decrease human coronary smooth muscle cell DNA synthesis. Arterioscler Thromb Vasc Biol. 1997, 17: 2088–95.

[61] Kohonen, T. Self-Organized formation of topologically correct feature maps. Biol. Cybern. 1982, 43: 59-69.

[62] Kohonen, T. Self-Organizing Maps. 3rd ed. Springer, 2001, Berlin, Germany.

[63] Kohonen, T. Kaski, S. Somervuo, P. Lagus, K. Oja, M. Paatero, V. Self-organizing map, Neurocomputing, 1998. 21: 113-122.

[64] Cocchi, M. Tonello, L. Bosi, S. Cremonesi, A. Castriota, F. Puri, B. Tsaluchidu, S. Platelet oleic acid as Ischemic Cardiovascular Disease marker. BMJ. 2007, Electronic letter to the editor.

[65] Cocchi, M. Tonello, L. Cappello, G. Bosi, S. Cremonesi, A. Castriota, F. Mercante, M. Tarozzi, G. Bochicchio, D. Della Casa, G. Caramia, G. Membrane platelet fatty acids: a model of biochemical characterisation of the ischemic cardiovascular disease, through an artificial neural network interpretation, Progr Nutr. 2008, 10, 1: 48-52.

[66] Cocchi, M. Tonello, L. Lercker, G. Platelet Stearic Acid in different population groups: biochemical and functional hypothesis. Nutr. clín. diet. hosp. 2009, 29: 34-45.

[67] Tonello, L. Cappello, G. Cocchi, M. "Nutritional Effects on Cardiovascular System", 3rd International Conference on Gravity and Cardiovascular System, 2006. INRC and CSV Italian Air Force (Pratica di Mare Air Force Base, November 13-15).

[68] Cocchi, M. Tonello, L. Platelets, Fatty Acids, Depression and Cardiovascular Ischemic Pathology, Progr Nutr. 2007, 9, 2: 94-104.

[69] Tiemeier, H. van Dijck, W. Hofman, A. Witteman, J.C.M. Stijnen, T. Breteler, M.M.B. Relationship between Atherosclerosis and Late-Life Depression. Arch Gen Psychiatry, 2004, 61: 369-376.

[70] Musselman, D.L. Evans, D.L. Nemeroff, C.B. The relationship of depression to cardiovascular disease epidemiology, biology, and treatment. Archives of General Psychiatry, 1998, 55: 580-592.

[71] Weyers, J. Colquhoun, D. For the OLIVE Study Group. A Mediterranean Diet (Med) Vs A Low Fat (Lf) Diet Improves Depression Independent of Cholesterol In Coronary Heart Disease Patients (CHD) June 29, 2000: Poster Abstracts.

[72] Cocchi, M. Mordenti, A.L. Merendi, F. Sardi, L. Tonello, L. Bochicchio, D. Faeti, V. Della Casa, G. Pig platelet fatty acids composition in different lipid treatments. LXI National Meeting SISVet (Salsomaggiore Terme, PR, Italy, Sep 26-29, 2007).

[73] Nichols, T.C. du Laney, T. Zheng, B. Bellinger Dwight, A. Nickols, G.A. Engleman, W. Clemmons, D.R. Reduction in Atherosclerotic Lesion Size in Pigs by aVb3 Inhibitors Is Associated With Inhibition of Insulin-Like Growth Factor-I–Mediated Signaling Circulation Research, 1999, 85: 1040-1045.

[74] Afri, M. Ehrenberg, B. Talmon, Y. Schmidt, J. Cohen, Y. Frimer, A.A. Active oxygen chemistry within the liposomial bilayer. Part III: Locating vitamin E, ubiquinol and ubiquinone and their derivatives in the lipid layer. Chem Phys Lipids, 2004, 3: 107-121.

[75] Gunstone, F.D. Harwood, J.L. Padley, F.B. The lipid handbook, Chapman & Hall Eds. London-New York, 1986, 453-457.

[76] Belitz H-D, Grosch W, Schieberle, P. Food Chemistry, Springer Verlag Ed., Berlin, Heidelberg, New York, London, Paris, Tokyo, 1987, 175.

[77] Wijesundera, C. Ceccato, C. Watkins, P. Fagan, P. Thienthong, N. Perlmutter, P. Docosahesaenoic acid is more stable to oxidation when located at the sn-2 position of triacylglycerol compared to sn-1(3). J Am Chem Soc. 2008, 85: 543-548.

[78] Sørensen A.D.M., Xu X., Zhang L., Kristensen J.B., Jacobsen C. (2010) Human Milk Fat Substitute from Butterfat: Production by Enzymatic Interesterification and Evaluation of Oxidative Stability. J. Am. Oil Chem. Soc., 87,185–194.

[79] La Rivista Italiana Delle Sostanze Grasse, 2002, Caratteristiche degli Oli e Grassi Vegetali. Suppl. n. 1-2.

[80] Bockish, M. Fats and Oils Handbook, 1998, AOCS Press, Champaign, Illinois, USA.

[81] International Olive Oil Council, IOOC Norms Refined olive oil, olive oil, olive-pomace-oil Purity criteria, www.oliveoilquotation.com/data/files/IOOC.

[82] Lercker, G. "I componenti minori delle sostanza grasse". Proceedings: IV Congresso Nazionale Acidi Grassi Polinsaturi Omega 3, CLA e Antiossidanti. Progr. Nutr. 2003, 5: 93-115.

[83] Regolamento (CEE) n. 2568/91 della Commissione dell'11 luglio 1991, relativo alle caratteristiche degli oli d'oliva e degli oli di sansa d'oliva nonché ai metodi ad essi attinenti, (G.U.C.E. L. 248 del 5 settembre 1991).

[84] Hove, E. L. Harris, P. L. Covitamin studies. V. The interrelation of a-tocopherol and essential unsaturated fat acids. J. Nutrition. 1946, 31: 699-713.

[85] Cocchi, M. Tonello, L. Bio molecular considerations in Major Depression and Ischemic Cardiovascular Disease. Central Nervous System Agents in Medicinal Chemistry. 2010, 10: 97-107.

Noninvasive Diagnostic Approach in Coronary Artery Disease

Chapter 3

Noninvasive Modalities for Coronary Angiography

Karthikeyan Ananthasubramaniam,
Sabha Bhatti and Abdul Hakeem

Additional information is available at the end of the chapter

1. Introduction

Optimal diagnostic quality non-invasive alternatives for visualization of the coronary arteries has been a major goal with the advent of newer cardiovascular imaging modalities such as coronary computed tomography angiography (CCTA) and magnetic resonance coronary angiography (MRCA). The challenges in imaging coronaries are obvious. The technology must be capable of visualizing arteries as small as 1.5 mm to delineate luminal and wall pathology which becomes challenging as many of the arteries are engulfed in tissue of similar composition. Coronary arteries exhibit rapid motion which poses major issues with blurring of images due to substantial limitations of temporal resolution. Invasive coronary angiography current enjoys the best temporal resolution (less than 20 msec) for real time visualization of coronaries and its branches but comes with its obvious limitations. CCTA has rapidly risen to this challenge and is already widely employed using 64 slice detector technology and is outstanding for exclusion of CAD with substantial advances in radiation reduction and speed of acquisition. MRCA has made significant improvements in technology which has made coronary imaging less challenging using navigator gating, whole heart imaging and using 3Tesla magnets, with the big advantage of no radiation and capability of non-contrast coronary imaging and most of all the promise of a true " one stop " comprehensive assessment. However, it is still suboptimal compared to CCTA as discussed subsequently in detail. This chapters aims to discuss MRCA and CCTA with regards to coronary imaging and compare and contrast both these imaging modalities with one another and also highlight some emerging comparisons of CCTA to invasive coronary luminal assessment technologies.

2. Magnetic Resonance Coronary Angiography (MRCA)

Introduction: MRCA has been performed for close to 20 years with numerous advances in technical and imaging aspects during this period although slower than CCTA explaining its slower adoption [1]. Initially 2 dimensional k space segmented imaging was done, but most centers now use whole heart free breathing navigator coronary MRI or targeted 3D imaging to enable better reconstruction capabilities. Published studies from experienced centers have shown excellent accuracy and superiority to conventional coronary angiography (CA) using 2 and 3 dimensional k space gradient echo MRCA (Table 1)[2]..

Although whole heart MRCA was initially performed with 4 channel cardiac coils and a parallel imaging factor of 2 [3, 4] it has been limited due longer acquisition times and image deterioration from diaphragmatic drift. Thirty two channel cardiac coils and higher parallel imaging factor of 4 [5] has potential for enhanced coronary imaging with whole heart MRCA. 3T MRCA gives higher signal to noise ratio (approximately 30%) but has its own limitations such as constructive/destructive interference in images causing dark and bright areas due to inherent in-homogeneities which worsen with strong magnetic fields [6]. Also specific absorption rates can increase upto 4 fold with 3T systems limiting use of certain imaging sequences. There are multiple components of MRCA namely cardiac triggering to suppress cardiac motion, respiratory motion suppression (navigator, breath hold) pre-pulses to enhance contrast noise ratio and image acquisition to enhance coronary arterial image quality. Overall image sequences for coronaries include black blood (fast spin echo and dual inversion) bright blood (segmented k space gradient echo and SSFP) all of which can be used either with 2D or 3D imaging.

Investigator	Technique	Respiratory Compensation	Number of Subjects	RCA	LM	LAD	LCX
Manning, 1993	2D GRE	BH	25	100%	96%	100%	76%
Pennell, 1993	2D GRE	BH	26	95%	95%	91%	76%
Duerinckx, 1994	2D GRE	BH	20	100%	95%	86%	77%
Sakuma, 1994	2D GRE cine	BH	18	100%	100%	100%	67%
Masui, 1995	2D GRE	BH	13	85%	92%	100%	92%
Davis, 1996	2D GRE	BH	33*	100%	100%	100%	100%
Li, 1993	3D GRE	Multiple Averages	14	100%	100%	86%	93%
Post, 1996	3D GRE	Retro Nav G	20	100%	100%	100%	100%
Wielopoiski, 1998	3D Seg EPI	BH	32	100%	100%	100%	100%
Botnar, 1999	3D GRE	Pro Nav G/C	13	97%	100%	100%	97%
Weber, 2003	3D SSFP	Pro Nav G/C	12	100%	100%	100%	100%

Abbreviations: BH, breath hold; GRE, gradient echo; LAD, left anterior descending coronary artery; LCX, left circumflex coronary artery; LM, left main coronary artery; PRO Nav GAC, prospective navigator gating with correction; RCA, right coronary artery; Retro Nav, retrospective navigator gating; Seg EPL, segmented EPI; SSFP, steady state free precession, 3D

Table 1. Successful visualization of native coronary arteries using 2 and 3 dimensional k space gradient echo MRCA [2].Obtained with permission

3. Challenges for MRCA

Achieving optimal spatial and temporal resolution, accurate motion compensation, wide anatomical coverage, and high signal and contrast to noise ratios are inherent challenges in MRCA. Improvement in one parameter occurs at the expense of another. Other factors that limit its widespread application in the acute setting include longer exam time, limited clinical monitoring in the scanner, device implants and other metallic objects that may need clearance prior to scanning.

Cardiac motion compensation deserves special mention. Since the heart moves due to both inherent motion and due to diaphragmatic movement and as the magnitude of this motion is greater than the diameter of the coronary vessels substantial blurring occurs if motion suppression techniques are not utilized [7]. A regular cardiac rhythm and reliable ECG gating is crucial for cardiac motion suppression techniques to work. Also time intervals of acquisition has to be determined in advance to plan the preparatory pulses which is a limitation. Acquisition is usually in mid-diastole due to least coronary motion and lasts for 50-150 milliseconds per cardiac cycle [8, 9].

As breath holds may be long during coronary imaging and impossible for some patients free breathing MRCA is an alternative and numerous correction techniques such as multiple averaging, chest wall bellows and navigator techniques have been attempted of which the latter is the most widely used [10].

MRCA Acquisition Methods:

1. **Pulse sequences:**

Pulse sequence design has evolved from black blood spin echo sequences to bright blood sequences such as gradient echo and steady state free precession (SSFP) imaging. Currently GRE is the chosen acquisition scheme in the majority of MRCA studies.

2. **Acquisition strategies:**

This includes k-space acquisition, contrast –enhanced (intrinsic and extrinsic) MRCA, 2D and 3D acquisitions. Despite many advances, the speed of acquisition and signal to noise ratio (SNR) remain limited. New strategies such as real time, parallel, time resolved and whole heart imaging have been developed.

1. CONVENTIONAL SPIN ECHO MRI: A spin echo signal results from a 90^0 RF pulse followed by a 180^0 pulse which refocuses the dephased spins up to a decay curve determined by the T2 relaxation time.

2. 2D SEGMENTED k SPACE GRADIENT ECHO MRI: The most widely available MRCA sequence is a 2D segmented k-space gradient echo acquisition usually performed in a single breath hold of fewer than 12 heartbeats. Thick slices and breath hold variability can limit registration of images from slice to slice however this sequence is adequate for applications such as evaluation for anomalous coronaries.

3. **3D MRI:** The use of navigator respiratory gating has given access to three-dimensional (3D) coronary magnetic resonance imaging techniques, allowing a 3D dataset to be obtained in a single acquisition. It provides higher spatial resolution and is less operator dependent. However, it relies on a reproducible respiratory pattern, which is not always present. Furthermore, 3D techniques are hampered by the saturation of blood signal, which decreases the signal to-noise ratio and the contrast of blood to myocardium.

4. **CONTRAST ENHANCED CORONARY MRI:** The use of interstitial paramagnetic contrast agents allows an improvement of signal and contrast. The disadvantage is the rapid leakage out of the intravascular space, amounting to 50% during the first pass. Multiple injections are necessary to cover the whole coronary artery tree. With the introduction of intravascular paramagnetic contrast agents [11, 12], the signal from blood no longer relies on inflow of blood but rather on the presence of the contrast agent itself. The imaging time can be prolonged with potential increased signal and in contrast, allowing a larger volume coverage and higher resolution.

5. **3T MRI:** Imaging at higher field strength can enhance signal-to-noise ratio (SNR) and enable higher spatial resolution. However, image quality may be hampered by increased susceptibility artifacts and RF inhomogeneity which may be addressed by shortening the TE and acquisition time. High-field imaging at 3 Tenhances spiral MRCA. A number of research groups already have demonstrated the feasibility of cardiac imaging at 7 T and beyond and have shown improved contrast between blood and epicardial fat, better coronary vessel sharpness, and increased blood signal intensity of the coronaries are obtained at 7 T than at 3 T [13].

Clinical Applications:

1. Anomalous coronary arteries:

C-MRA provides a 3D spatial relationship to great vessels, allowing evaluation of the origin and course of anomalous coronary arteries. Accurate delineation of proximal course has been shown with a sensitivity of 88-100% and specificity of 100% [14-19] MRI can often provide a definitive diagnosis in patients in whose X ray angiography is inconclusive. See Table 2

Investigator	Number of patients	Correctly Classified Anomalous Vessels
McConnell, 1995	15	14 (93%)
Post, 1995	19	19 (100%)
Vilegen, 1997	12	11 (92%)
Taylor, 2000	25	24 (96%)
Bunce, 2003	26	26 (100%)
Razmi, 2001	12	12 (100%)

Table 2. Anomalous coronary assessment by MRCA.[2] (reproduced with permission)

2. Coronary Artery Disease:

Clinical studies have produced variable results. Kim et al [20] performed the first multicenter trial in 109 patients with suspected CAD. Overall sensitivity and specificity was 93 and 42%, respectively. 84% of coronary segments were of diagnostic quality. Table 1 shows the comparative sensitivities of MRCA to CA. An example of MRCA coronary artery delineation is shown in Figures 1A and 1B

Sakuma et al [21] evaluated over 130 patients with significant CAD and found an overall accuracy of 87%, per patient sensitivity of 82% and specificity of 90%

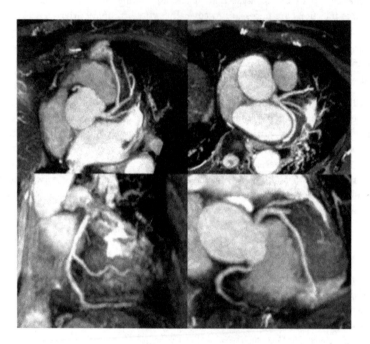

Figure 1. Sliding partial MIP images of 3 T whole heart coronary MRA acquired with a patient-specific narrow acquisition window (50 ms) in the cardiac cycle Journal of Cardiovascular Magnetic Resonance **Vol.** 11 **Issue** Suppl 1 2009-01-2

4. Coronary Computed Tomoraphy Angiography (CCTA)

Introduction: CCTA has been rapidly adopted in a short time span by institutions across the world as the most widely used anatomic noninvasive imaging modality for coronary artery assessment. A major reason for this is the existing wide use of CT for non-cardiac applications and most institutions have access to a CT scanner. Thus, investing in a state of the art

CT scanner serves multiple purposes and makes financial sense with opportunity for cardiac and non-cardiac use. Although initially limited to electron beam scanners in the 1980's where imaging of the heart arteries took several seconds and processing several hours, with the advent of multi-detector coronary computed CT technology (MDCT or multi slice (MSCT)) in the late 1990's, rapid advancement in scanner technology has enabled rapid whole heart acquisitions in a few seconds. With such scanners post processing capabilities on a 3D dataset is usually achievable in about 15-20 minutes.

CCTA requires high temporal resolution to minimize motion artifacts caused by cardiac motion and breathing. This requires a fast gantry rotation with multiple detectors. Because the coronaries are seen best when there is least motion, the diastolic phase is most optimal for imaging and thus the temporal resolution must be less than the length of the diastolic phase. High spatial resolution is also necessary to allow imaging of the coronary arteries which are small and tortuous. At present, 64-detector row CT systems are the most widely employed platform for performing CCTA. The 64 detectors allow an x-,y- axis (in-plane) spatial resolution of near 0.4mm and the z-axis spatial resolution or slice thickness is almost 0.6mm. Fast contiguous coverage of the heart is required to allow imaging of the entire heart in one breath hold. This requires the multi-slice helical CT technique, each slice of the heart is collected in one or more heartbeats. There is a 30%-50% overlap between each slice. The scan must be triggered to the heartbeat to allow gating so that imaging in multiple slices occurs across multiple heartbeats. Table 3 below, is a summary of the state of art 64 slice CT scanners with their various technical specifications [22].

Scanner	X-ray sources, n	Detector rows, n	Detector-row x-axis dimension, mm*	Total nominal beam width, mm	Fastest gantry rotation time, second	Temporal resolution for each cross-sectional image, second[†]
GE Discovery CT750 HD	1	64	0.625	40	0.35	0.175
Hitachi SCENARIA	1	64	0.625	40	0.35	0.175
Philips Brilliance iCT	1	128[‡]	0.625	80	0.27	0.135
Siemens SOMATOM Definition FLASH	2 (95° apart)	64[‡]	0.6	40	0.28	0.075
Toshiba Aquilion ONE	1	320	0.5	160	0.35	0.175

*Values measured at scanner isocenter.
[†]Values do not reflect the use of multisegment reconstruction.
[‡]Uses z-axis flying focal spot to sample each detector twice per rotation.

Table 3. Reproduced under permission from [22]

Patient preparation:

On the day of the test, patients should take medications as scheduled especially betablockers. Metformin should be avoided because of the potential adverse effects when used concomitantly with iodinated contrast agents. Phosphodiesterase inhibitors should be avoided 48 hours before a CCTA because nitrates are needed to dilate the coronary arteries. Premedication with mucomyst and hydration are recommended if the creatinine is elevated. If a contrast allergy is present, premedication with steroids and antihistamines is required. A right antecubital IV that is at least 18-gauge is preferred. If heart rate is not low enough with oral beta-blockers, IV beta-blockers may be useful.

Data Acquisition:

Two types of ECG gating are possible, prospective and retrospective. Prospective is where the scanner emits radiation only at a predefined point after the R wave. Mid-diastole occurs at 70-75% of the R-R interval and during this time in the cardiac cycle, there is minimum amount of motion enabling better coronary imaging. The CT beam is off during all other points in the cycle. This requires a regular heart rate and is the preferred method of imaging because of the low radiation dose. In retrospective triggering a continuous heart scan is utilized. Imaging is performed throughout systole and diastole. Left ventricular function data is hence available. This method of gating is used if the patient's heart rate is irregular or not low enough for 64 slice CT scanners. Figure 2 below shows the different modes of CCCT acquisition [22].

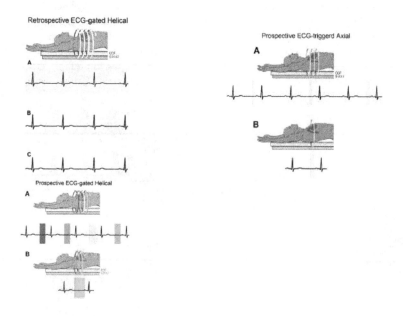

Figure 2. Reproduced under permission from [22]

Radiation Exposure: Reported CTA effective radiation dose is higher than many other cardiac diagnostic procedures as described by the International Commission on Radiological Protection (ICRP) 60 [23]. The rapid expansion of CCCTA magnifies the importance of dose reduction within the population. The clinical acceptance of CCCTA will partially depend on the radiation exposure and its consequences, particularly if it is going to be used at an earlier stage of CAD detection. Some commonly used dose reduction strategies include:

1. Restricting scan field to anatomy of interest (~1 cm above left main to ~1 cm below heart)

2. Reducing peak mAs based on body size (non-contrast scout films may be used to estimate image noise)

3. Using ECG dependant current modulation with lowest mAs during systole. Narrowing the width of the peak mAs phase

4. Reducing kV to 100 if body Wt is <85 kg

5. Use prospective gating if available.

With regards to radiation exposure numerous algorithms and acquisition techniques have been developed as discussed previously to reduce exposure specifically prospective triggered acquisition [24] and high pitch acquisition with dual source CCTA [25].

5. Limitations

There are several limitations with CCTA. Patients unable to cooperate with scanning instructions should be considered for other imaging modalities. Uncontrollable arrhythmias can result in significant motion artifacts and multiple uninterpretable coronary segments. Contraindications to iodinated contrast use include pregnancy, prior severe/anaphylactic contrast reaction and renal insufficiency (but end-stage renal disease is not a contraindication) for contrast-induced nephropathy. Certain conditions should raise concerns for the use of pre-scan beta-blocker (chronic obstructive pulmonary disease/asthma, decompensated heart failure, and advanced atrioventricular block) and nitroglycerin (severe aortic stenosis, hypertrophic cardiomyopathy, recent phosphodiesterase-5 inhibitor use). Metallic objects such as pacemakers, intra-cardiac defibrillator leads, prosthetic valves cause beam-hardening and streaking artifact over adjacent coronary arteries. Dense concentric coronary calcification causes a blooming artifact, which often leads to overestimation of degree of stenosis.

Clinical Applications:

Most Important Appropriate indications for CCTA

Chest pain evaluation after an uninterpretable or equivocal stress test
Chest pain evaluation in patients with an intermediate probability, an uninterpretable EKG and unable to exercise
Acute chest pain evaluation, an intermediate pretest probability, no EKG changes, and serial enzymes negative
Suspected coronary anomalies in symptomatic patients
Coronary evaluation in new onset heart failure

Table 4.

1. **Anomalous coronary arteries:** CTA provides a 3D spatial relationship to great vessels, allowing evaluation of the origin and course of anomalous coronary arteries in a non–invasive manner. It is the "gold standard" test for evaluating anomalous coronary arteries and has the highest level of appropriateness use for this indication.

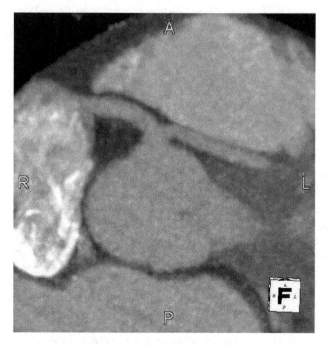

Figure 3. 40 year old male with syncope during exercise. CCTA shows anomalous left main coronary artery take off from right coronary cusp between aorta and RVOT

2. **Coronary artery disease**

i.   **Detection of Coronary Stenosis:** With ongoing technical development, the diagnostic performance of CT with respect to detection and quantification of obstructive CAD is steadily improving. The confidence and accuracy to assess stenosis is better in larger branches and in the absence of extensive coronary calcification. For the assessment of individual coronary segments, the sensitivity to detect significant coronary artery stenosis ranges between 64-99%, the specificity between 84- 98%, with pooled average sensitivity of 87% and specificity of 96%. The positive predictive value is approximately 80% whereas the negative predictive value has been consistently high in all the studies with a pooled average of 98%. Calcified coronary disease causes blooming artifacts, which increases apparent stenosis severity of a lesion. The ability to quantify coronary stenosis severity has been modest compared to invasive angiography given the limited spatial resolution of CT and blooming artifacts of calcified lesions. There are numerous single-center [26-34] and three multicenter studies [35-37] using different scanner technologies (Table 4) [35-37] in symptomatic patients with suspected CAD.

						Per-patient base analysis	
Author	Year	Patients	CAD prevalence (%)	Sensitivity	Specificity	Positive predictive value	Negative predictive value
Budoff et al.	2008	230	25	95	83	64	99
Miller et al.	2008	291	56	85	90	91	83
Meijboom et al.	2008	360	68	99	64	86	97

CAD, coronary artery disease.

Table 5. Adapted with permission from Chang et al [38].

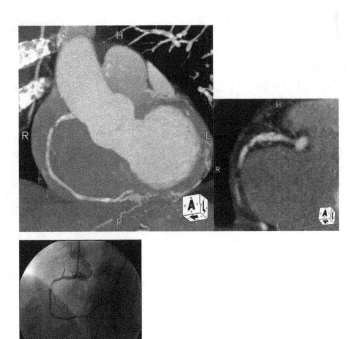

Figure 4. CCTA of a 60 year old smoker with atypical chest pain and sub-maximal negative stress echo. Thick maximum intensity projection (MIP) images and multiplanar reconstruction images (MPR) are shown showing focal high grade stenosis in proximal-mid RCA accompanied by scattered calcified plaques throughout RCA, Coronary angiogram was performed confirming CCTA findings.

ii.   **Stents:** CCTA is not optimal for the evaluation of coronary stents because the spatial resolution is not quite good enough to visualize the intrastent lumen, thus should not be routinely used for the evaluation of coronary stents. Small stents tend to cause blooming and beam hardening issues leading to poor delineation of lumen. Lack of contrast in lumen is a sign of in-stent restenosis. Currently, larger stents >3.5-4.0 mm may be adequately assessed [39].

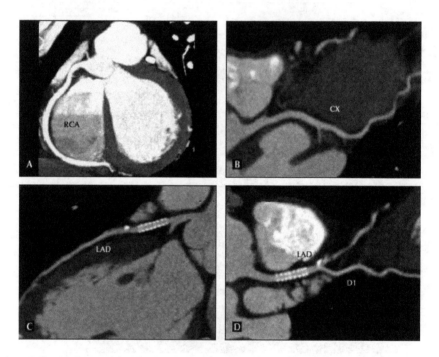

Figure 5. Shows multiplanar reformats of the left anterior descending coronary artery with clear visualization of patent stents and normal right and left circumflex coronary arteries. Reproduced from Cademartiri et al [39].

iii.   **Bypass Graft Analysis:** CCTA may be used to assess bypass graft patency as well as to evaluate the patient undergoing repeat bypass surgery. In repeat bypass surgery CCTA is utilized to identify the location of a previously utilized graft. Clips may often create challenges in assessing bypass grafts because of beam hardening artifact and their potential to obscure the graft lumen or anastomosis point. Below is an example of a 3d surface rendering of patient with prior coronary artery bypass surgery (Figure 6) [40]. The saphenous vein graft (SVG) to the right coronary artery is seen taking off from the aorta and inserting into the RCA. The origins of 2 other SVG are also noted adjacent to the SVG to RCA going to the left coronary system. The maximum intensity projection reveals a significant stenosis in the insertion site of the SVG to RCA [40].

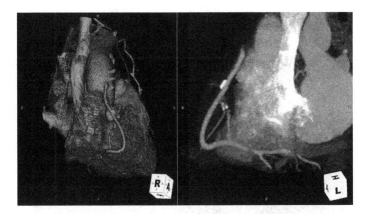

Figure 6.

3. Role of CCTA in Emergency Department:

A significant amount of money is wasted on inappropriate chest pain evaluations and admissions. Given CTA's high NPV, the test would most benefit the intermediate-probability patients in the ED. By using CTA, hospitalization could be avoided in patients presenting to ED with chest pain. Logistic issues such as ED scanner availability and 24 hour expertise in CTA interpretation limit use of CTA in most institutions. Triple rule out protocols have been developed and studied to rule out coronary disease, pulmonary embolism and aortic dissection [27, 41, 42]. These are however not used widely due to logistic issues and since often one or more of these 3 etiologies can be ruled out clinically. A recent meta analysis by Samad et al [43] synthesized data from 9 studies involving 1349 patients presenting to the emergency room with suspected acute coronary syndrome (ACS). Endpoint was the diagnostic performance of CTA for ACS. The bivariate summary estimate of sensitivity of CTA for ACS diagnosis was 95% (95% CI 88-100) and specificity was 87% (95% CI 83-92), yielding a negative likelihood ratio of 0.06 (95% CI 0-0.14) and positive likelihood ratio of 7.4 (95% CI 4.8-10). Based on this meta analysis of all the clinical studies, coronary CTA with its high sensitivity and a low negative likelihood ratio of 0.06, is effective in ruling out the presence of ACS in low to intermediate risk patients presenting to the ED with acute chest pain. More recently the role of CCTA in ER has been studied in 2 important randomized trials the ACRIN-PA [44] and the ROMICAT-2. Both studies showed that CCTA has an outstanding negative predictive value with low subsequent event rates although conventional management including stress testing also achieved comparable results. There was shorter length of stay and quicker discharge directly from ED in CCTA arm although costs were the same between CCTA and conventional testing in ROMICAT-2. Also radiation doses and downstream testing were higher in CCTA arm in ROMICAT-2 [45]. An important point with regards to use of CCTA in ED is that although a zero calcium score makes obstructive CAD highly unlikely as a cause of chest pain it is now clear that young patients (age < 50, smokers) may present with non-calcified obstructive disease and thus should not be triaged based on a negative calcium score alone (see Figure 7 below)

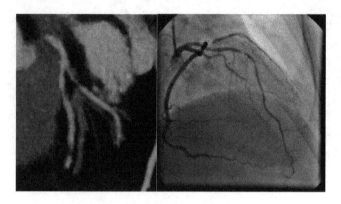

Figure 7. 30 year old male with history of 15 pack history of smoking, cocaine abuse presents with intermittent substernal pressure of 3 days duration. Coronary CT was done. Non-contrast scan showed zero calcium score but CCTA showed high grade stenosis in the LAD and diagonal. The image on left is a view of the mid LAD showing mainly non-calcified obstructive plaque. Coronary angiography confirms high grade LAD.

4.   Role of CCTA in Assessing Etiology of Cardiomyopathy

It is extremely important to define the etiology of cardiomyopathies to enable appropriate management and therapies. CCTA can be of critical importance to rule out ischemic cardiomyopathy in a non-invasive manner. CCTA has immensely robust accuracy at evaluating the proximal vascular bed with accuracy approaching almost 97-100%. This attribute becomes most relevant in the context of ischemic cardiomyopathy which per the standardized definition proposed by Felker et al [46][Patients with 75% stenosis of left main or proximal LAD, patients with 75% stenosis of two or more epicardial vessels] yields a very high diagnostic odds ratio for ischemic cardiomyopathy. Several studies have evaluated the diagnostic accuracy of CCTA in comparison with invasive angiography. We performed a meta analysis of all 6 studies involving 452 patients with cardiomyopathy of undetermined cause who underwent CTA. All patients also underwent diagnostic invasive angiography. The pooled summary estimate of sensitivity was 98% and specificity 97% yielding a negative likelihood ratio of 0.06 for ischemic cardiomyopathy. The receiver operator curve analysis showed a robust discriminate diagnostic accuracy of ischemic etiology with an AUC of 0.99(Figure 8). With a pooled sensitivity of 98%, an ischemic etiology of left ventricular systolic dysfunction can be accurately "ruled out" with CTA (>16 slices). A negative study hence essentially excludes the presence of ischemic cardiomyopathy. A positive CTA effectively "rules in" the probability that an underlying cardiomyopathy could be related to significant epicardial coronary stenosis. Hence, CTA can be considered as an invaluable imaging modality for evaluating patients with left ventricular dysfunction of a suspected ischemic etiology [47].

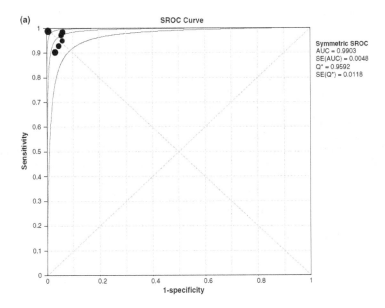

Figure 8. Diagnostic accuracy of CCTA for ischemic cardiomyopathy. Adapted with permission from Bhatti et al [47].

6. Comparison of MSCT angiography and Invasive angiography

Since the first report of Moshage et al over 17 years ago [48], numerous studies and meta analyses have been published confirming the superior diagnostic performance of MSCT in comparison with invasive angiography as the reference standard.. The largest meta analysis to date collated data from 89 studies with 7516 patients [49]. Bivariate analysis yielded a mean sensitivity and specificity were 97.2% (95% CI, 96.2% to 98.0%) and 87.4% (CI, 84.5% to 89.8%) for CT. Negative likelihood ratio was 0.03 (0.02-0.04) whereas the positive likelihood ratio was modest at 7.7(6.2-9.5) area under the curve was 0.98 (CI, 0.96 to 0.99) for CT. The resulting sensitivity of 98.1% for scanners with more than 16 detector rows was significantly higher ($P < 0.050$) than that for scanners with a maximum of 16 rows (95.6%). The high negative predictive value of CTA best suites it as an effective rule-out test for significant CAD.

Despite the use of newer generation scanners (>64 slice), coronary calcification remains the Achilles heel of CTA. A recent analysis from the CORE 64 study demonstrated that the robust AUC of CTA (0.93) significantly decreased to (0.81) in patients with calcium score >600 [50]. Furthermore, the negative predictive value of CTA decreased from 0.93 in patients with Calcium score <100 to 0.75 in patients with calcium score >100. High pretest probability of CAD and high calcium score negatively impacts the diagnostic performance of CTA and must be carefully considered in test selection.

7. Prognostic value

Whereas the diagnostic accuracy of CCTA has been rigorously established, increasing number of studies have also evaluated the prognostic value of CCTA. A recent meta analysis included eighteen studies involving 9,592 patients with a median follow-up of 20 months for adverse cardiac events [51]. The authors computed a pooled annualized event MACE rate of 8.8% for obstructive (any vessel with >50% luminal stenosis) disease versus 0.17% per year for normal CCTA (p < 0.05) and 3.2% versus 0.15% for death or MI (p < 0.05) Figure 9. Furthermore, the pooled negative likelihood ratio for MACE after normal CCTA findings was 0.008 (95% CI: 0.0004 to 0.17, p < 0.001). Patients with a normal CTA can hence be confidently reassured given a very low risk of death, MI or revascularization fairly comparable to an otherwise healthy population(<1%). Furthermore, the low event rate for normal CTA (0.16%) is comparable to other well established non invasive risk stratification modalities including stress echocardiography (0.45%) and myocardial perfusion stress imaging (0.54%). CTA has hence emerged as a well established clinical tool that carries not only robust diagnostic accuracy but also has powerful predictive accuracy as well [51].

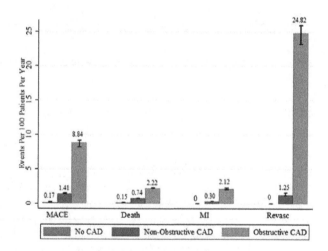

Figure 9. Adapted with permission from Hulten et al [51]

8. Physiological significance of stenoses identified by CTA

That, coronary angiography is merely a "luminogram" and does not provide much insight into the hemodynamic significance of a stenotic lesion, is a fact that has been rigorously established for the past two decades. This well-recognized limitation has been documented repeatedly by intravascular ultrasound imaging and stress testing. It has been known that coronary angiography often leads to overestimation of the functional significance of epicardial coronary stenoses. In this regard, fractional flow reserve (FFR) has emerged as a powerful catheter based tool that provides robust information about the functional severity of the lesion. FFR calculated from coronary pressure measurement, is a reliable, invasive index to indicate if a stenosis is ischemia-related and can be determined in the catheterization laboratory in a simple and rapid way. By taking the ratio of the coronary pressure measured distal to the stenosis to aortic pressure as the normal perfusion pressure (distal coronary pressure/aortic pressure) and obtaining these measurements when the microvascular resistance was minimal and assumed to be constant (that is, at maximal hyperemia), the percentage of normal coronary flow, or a fraction of normal flow (i.e., FFR), can be calculated. FFR has a uniform normal value of 1.0 for every patient and every coronary artery; it is not dependent on changes in heart rate, blood pressure, or contractility; it accounts for collateral flow; and it has a sharp threshold value to indicate inducible ischemia: FFR < 0.75 always indicates inducible ischemia; FFR > 0.80 excludes ischemia in 90% of the cases [15, 17-20, 23, 46, 52-54]. The grey zone is very limited, which is important for clinical decision making in an individual patient. Coronary pressure measurements can be easily performed by a pressure wire, with almost identical mechanical properties as normal guide wires, and barely prolong the procedure, even when multiple vessels are interrogated. The ischemic threshold of FFR has been replicated independently with different noninvasive functional tests in numerous studies (including exercise electrocardiography, dobutamine stress echocardiography, and MPI) as well as alongside one another in the same population. An FFR >0.75 identified coronary stenoses in patients with inducible myocardial ischemia with high sensitivity (88%), specificity (100%), positive predictive value (100%), and overall accuracy (93%). FFR has a high reproducibility and low intra-individual variability. Several randomized clinical trials including DEFER, FAME and now FAME II have established the prognostic utility of FFR.Consequently, now, measurement of FFR during invasive coronary angiography is the gold standard for identifying coronary artery lesions that cause ischemia and improves clinical decision-making for revascularization.

Similar limitations of stenoses especially in the intermediate range (50-70%) are widely seen in CT angiograms. This poses both diagnostic and therapeutic challenges. Meijboom et al [55] evaluated 89 lesions in 79 patients with stable angina. Lesion correlation with invasive angiography was performed and FFR of stenoses was measured. The authors demonstrated very poor correlation between CTA and invasive coronary angiography with hemodynamically significant stenosis (FFR<0.75); diagnostic accuracy 64% for FFR <0.8 and 49% for FFR< 0.75. CTA overestimated the functional significance of coronary stenoses (poor specificity/high false positive rate) even after excluding segments with high calcification and coronary motion. Hence patients with intermediate stenoses on CTA require further evaluation by either FFR evaluation of stress testing.

Recently, evaluation of FFR from CCTA data (FFRCT) has been proposed as a noninvasive method for identifying ischemic lesions. This employs the concept of computational fluid dynamics (CFD) Koo et al [56] correlated FFR from CT data with invasive FFR in 103 patients (159 vessels) in a prospective multicenter DISCOVER-FLOW (Diagnosis of Ischemia-Causing Stenoses Obtained via Noninvasive Fractional Flow Reserve) study. On a per-vessel basis, the accuracy, sensitivity, specificity, positive predictive value, and negative predictive value were 84.3%, 87.9%, 82.2%, 73.9%, 92.2%, respectively, for FFRCT and were 58.5%, 91.4%, 39.6%, 46.5%, 88.9%, respectively, for CCTA stenosis yielding an AUC of 0.9 for FFR CT and 0.75 for CTA. There was fair correlation between invasive FFR and FFRCT (r = 0.717, p < 0.001) although FFR Ct had slight underestimation (0.022 ± 0.116, p = 0.016). The results of the larger 285 patient DEFACTO trial comparing CT FFR and invasive FFR are awaited later this year and would further consolidate the role of non invasive FFR in the evaluation of intermediate coronary lesions see on CTA.

9. Complimentary role of CTA in guiding complex PCI like Chronic total occlusion (CTOs)

The unprecedented spatial resolution and 3D reconstruction of the epicardial coronary vessels has led to its role as an indispensable tool in guiding complex coronary interventions including recanalizing chronic total occlusions (CTO); the most challenging subset of complex coronary lesions. The display of CTA images as a 3D roadmap, side-by-side with live angiography images is instrumental in providing the interventional team access to the occluded channel. Furthermore, synchronization of the CTA image orientation with the C-arm, allows for selection of the ideal treatment projection angle without additional contrast medium or radiation exposure. Several studies have validated the use of CTA in guiding CTO intervention [57].

10. Diagnostic accuracy of CTA for in-stent restenosis

Despite the introduction of drug eluting stents, instent restenosis (ISR) from neointimal hyperplasia remains a real issue. For patients with recurrent chest pain following stent implantation, invasive coronary angiography is often performed to evaluate the presence of ISR. However, the need for a noninvasive alternative approach for ISR detection is more desirable. The experience with older generation CTA systems (4 and 16 slice) in evaluation of ISR was very disappointing largely related to motion and blooming artifacts. The improved spatial and temporal resolution with 64,128 and 256 slice scanners seems to have ameliorated those limitations. Carrabba et al [58] performed a meta analysis of nine studies involving 598 participants with 978 stents evaluated for ISR with CTA (64 slice) using invasive coronary angiography as the reference standard. More than 60% of the studied stents were >3 mm in diameter. Approximately 10% of the stents were unassessable. The pooled sensitivity and specificity of CTA was 86% (95% CI 80-91%) and 93%(95% CI 91-95%) respectively yielding an AUC of 0.94 for per stent analysis. The calculated positive and negative predictive values were 70.4% and 97.2%, respectively. CTA can hence 64-MDCT can hence reliably rule out ISR and further evaluation by means of invasive coronary angiography can be avoided.

Caution is still advised for smaller stents and the fact that almost 10% of the studies were still uninterpretable despite the use of 64 detector scanners.

11. Comparison of coronary computed tomography angiography and magnetic resonance coronary angiography

This section aims to compare the techniques of coronary computed tomography angiography (CCTA) with magnetic resonance coronary angiography (MRCA) from the standpoint of coronary and cardiac imaging.

12. Comparison of technical aspects CCTA to MRCA

Currently the majority of the institutions utilize 64 slice technology (in-plane spatial resolution of 0.4 x 0.4 mm with a slice thickness of 0.6 mm and a 360° gantry rotation in about 330 milliseconds). More recently dual source CCTA technology has pushed the envelope further and has delivered a temporal resolution of 70-83 msec with an in plane resolution of 0.4 mm [59]. Furthermore, 256 and 320 slice CT- scanners are available in limited institutions across the world which can image the entire heart in 1 beat thus obviating many limitations with current 64 slice scanners such as irregular heart rhythm, breath hold issues and opening options for perfusion CCCTA imaging.

The tremendous advantages that CCTA holds over MRCA with such high spatial resolution relates to: 1. ability to visualize small diameter vessels including distal coronary branches, 2. increased ability to quantify calcium and reduce blooming artifacts, 3. better visualization of stents, and 4. better plaque morphology assessment. The temporal resolution advances in CCTA has enabled: 1. enhanced ability to freeze cardiac motion, 2. additional reconstruction capabilities within cardiac cycle, and 3. reduced scan time.

The obvious disadvantages of CCTA compared to MRCA are: 1. radiation exposure which depending on the scanner, mode of acquisition and protocol modifications can range from 1 milliseivert to > 15 milliseiverts[60, 61], 2. use of iodinated contrast which could pose issues for patients with underlying renal dysfunction, and 3. need for slow heart rates which require use of beta-blockers.

13. One stop shop imaging : MRCA versus CCTA

A very attractive advantage with MRCA is that it can combined with detailed cardiac MRI exam to provide a "one stop shop" assessment is easily achievable where coronary disease, valves, stress/rest perfusion for ischemia and viability and overall cardiac and adjacent thoracic and extra-thoracic anatomy can be all studied without concern for nephrotoxic contrast or repetitive exposure to radiation. Furthermore, imaging sequences or views can easily be repeated. Thus, a hybrid anatomic and functional assessment is clinically feasible at present in centers with experience with MRCA. With CCTA, valves and ventricular function assessment comes at the cost of higher radiation exposure as retrospective triggered acquisition is needed. CT perfusion imaging for ischemia and viability is still not well validated compared to cardiac MRI but has been performed for both viability [62, 63] and perfusion [64, 65] and is being tested against SPECT in ongoing clinical trials. Promising new studies with CCTA with lower radiation doses encompassing a complete anatomical-functional assessment compared to traditional SPECT imaging has been published recently [66] but this aspect of CCTA is not ready for clinical use. Although MRCA does offer high temporal resolution, good spatial resolution, high soft tissue contrast and the ability to generate any three dimensional image without need for ionizing radiation it is much more challenging to perform as it requires selection of the correct pulse sequences and each pulse sequence needs many parallel slices or slab volumes to cover the entire heart. Free breathing MRCA acquisitions can take 5-15 minutes compared to a few seconds with current 64-320 slice CCTA. Spatial resolution of CCTA is superior to MRCA (0.4 to -0.6 mm with CCTA compared to 1.5 mm with MRCA). The disadvantage for MRCA compared to CCTA in terms of speed of acquisition is difficult to overcome although breath hold MRCA may offer some improvement in time required for acquisition compared to free breathing techniques [67]. The temporal resolution of CCTA is limited by the gantry rotation speed and hence cannot be altered. On the contrary free breathing MRCA temporal resolution can be flexibly determined using imaging parameters. The acquisition window position and the length within the RR interval can be individually set [68]. This is an important advantage with MRCA.

14. Diagnostic accuracy of CCTA versus MRCA for CAD

The diagnostic accuracy of CCTA is well established with it outstanding negative predictive value (97.2%) and moderate-to good positive predictive value (87.4%) based on cumulative data from 89 studies of 7519 patients(69). This compares much more favorably to MRCA which has a sensitivity of 87.1% and specificity of 70.3 % based on 20 studies of 989 patients [69]. Furthermore, in patients suspected of CAD or with acute disease at presentation, CCTA has an outstanding negative likelihood ratio of 0.03(0.02-0.04) and 0.06(0.02-0.19) respectively [69]. A meta-analysis of CCTA versus MRCA [49] and a recent study comparing state of art 64 slice CCTA to 32 channel 3T MRCA [70] both concluded that although both modalities performed well for CAD detection CCTA outperformed MRCA. Furthermore CCTA was completed in 13.9+/= 1.1 sec compared to 17 +/- 4.7 minutes for MRCA [70]. The expert consensus document on "appropriate" use of CT and MRI imaging published in 2006 gave an appropriate indication for CCTA to rule out significant CAD in patients with chest pain and intermediate likelihood of CAD. On the contrary the document gave a recommendation of "inappropriate" for MRCA for the same indication [71]. This reflects the lack of adequate data demonstrating the feasibility and accuracy for MRCA on a practical level across many institutions.

15. Assessment of coronary anomalies and aneurysms: CCTA versus MRCA

One important indication where MRCA could be very helpful is imaging for anomalous coronaries in children and young adults where exposure to radiation from CCTA is undesirable [72]. Coronary arteries in MRCA can be imaged without nephrotoxic contrast administration. The high T2/T1 signal in steady state free precession imaging (SSFP) acts as a natural contrast agent providing coronary lumen definition [73]. However, SSFP imaging has greater susceptibility to artifacts and newer sequences such as fast low angle shots (FLASH) show better imaging characteristics at 3.0T compared to SSFP [74] also showing a 50% reduction in scan time [75]. CCTA offers outstanding spatial resolution and is the widely preferred technique at least in adults to evaluate anomalous coronaries as long as there are no inherent contraindications to its use. ACC/AHA appropriate use guidelines for CCTA /MRI [71] gives CCTA and MRCA an " appropriate" indication score with CCTA receiving a higher score of 9 compared to MRCA which also receives a high score of 8. MRCA may also be used for serial follow-up of coronary aneurysms which can be a sequelae of Kawasaki disease particularly in adolescents and young adults who otherwise may need repeated angiography.[76, 77] CCTA again is excellent to delineate these aneurysms but suffers from limitations of repetitive radiation exposure.

16. Comparison of Technical Challenges in Imaging for CCTA and MRCA

16.1. Motion artifact issues : CCTA versus MRCA

Motion artifacts pose a significant problem with both MRCA and CCTA. In MRCA this can be intrinsic related to cardiac contraction /relaxation or extrinsic attributable to diaphragm and chest wall movement during respiration [35]. Furthermore, MRCA requires expertise to perform and interpret and is currently limited largely to academic centers with a dedicated 1.5 or a 3T cardiac magnet at least in North America. In CCTA motion artifacts are related to patient motion and respiratory based artifact (as CCTA imaging is during breath hold). In contrast 64 slice CCTA is available in most large institutions and practices and the training and interpretation process is much more feasible for physicians desiring to practice this technology.

16.2. Calcification issues: CCTA versus MRCA

Calcification of coronary arteries is seen in at least 50-70% of patients with atherosclerotic plaques [78]. Calcium poses a significant limitation for accuracy of CCTA due to blooming/beam hardening artifacts compromising lumen assessment [79]. However it is not a limitation for MRCA for assessing the lumen of the coronary arteries as MRI does not have issues with beam hardening or blooming. Thus lumen visualization is not compromised [80]. The flip side of this is the added advantage of detection of coronary calcium during the non-contrast portion of CCTA which serves both to diagnose atherosclerosis [81] and in its absence make obstructive CAD highly unlikely both in asymptomatic patients and in patient with suspected cardiac etiology of chest pain [82, 83]. Coronary calcium also provides powerful prognostic information and is incremental in risk assessment beyond traditional risk scores like Framingham risk scores [84]. Furthermore, identifying substantial calcium may also help in decision making for the physician as the CCTA portion of the test could be cancelled and more definitive testing towards significance of underlying lesion could be pursued wither with stress testing or angiography. MRCA lack this important " heads up" diagnostic advantage that CCTA possess as part of its armamentarium due to its inability to image calcium. More recently some investigators have tried to exploit the different capabilities of CCTA and MRCA by combining both technologies in patients with significant calcification. In a small study of 18 patients who underwent 64 slice CCTA, 3D free breathing MRCA and coronary angiography, MRCA had better diagnostic image quality and performed better in detection of obstructive CAD in coronary segments with focal rather than diffuse calcification and overall performed better than CCTA in detecting significant CAD in patients with high calcium scores [80].

17. Imaging bypass grafts and stents: CCTA versus MRCA

CCTA is an outstanding modality for imaging bypass grafts. In a study by Liu and colleagues [85] 228 patients underwent 64 slice CCTA to evaluate diagnostic accuracy of CCTA for bypass graft disease. The sensitivity, specificity, positive negative predictive value and overall accuracy were reported at an impressive 93.3%, 98.1%, 93.3%, 98.1%, and 97.7 % respectively. Major disadvantages include higher contrast dose, increased radiation from longer scanning to cover the anatomy of origin and course of grafts and artifacts related to clips from surgery. The anastamotic sites in particular can sometimes be challenging to evaluate. In comparison, in a study by Langerak et al,[86] MRCA showed a sensitivity and specificity of 83 and 100% for graft occlusion,82%, and 88% for graft stenosis >/= 50% and 73% and 80% for graft stenosis >/= 70%. MRCA also suffers from signal void artifacts from metallic implants, clips, etc. In addition it seems to perform inferior to CCTA in consistently identifying severely diseased yet patent vessels [86] making its widespread applicability for bypass graft evaluation less feasible. Furthermore even though CCTA has limitations with radiation the population with CABG are older and hence the lifetime risk of cancer is less of a concern. Newer generation 64 slice CCTA has also shown promise in imaging stent lumen although stents less than 3 mm tend to cause unacceptable degree of lumen visualization and blooming artifacts (highest with tantalum stents and lowest with titanium and nitinol based alloys) and CCTA is not recommended below this size. A recent study on coronary stent patency with CCTA showed a promising 89% sensitivity and 95% specificity [87]. MRCA data with stents is limited but the stainless steel composition of stents make imaging challenging as in-stent integrity and persistent assessment can be compromised. The attractive force and local heart generated with stent imaging at 1.5 T and 3T is not a major issue the local susceptibility artifacts can be a big problem [88, 89]. This is less of problem with tantalum compared to stainless steel stents. In the USA both Cypher and Taxus Liberte stents are approved for imaging with MRI immediately after implantation.

18. Contrast issues: CCTA versus MRCA

CCTA has to utilize iodinated contrast agents between 80-120 ml for opacification of coronary vessels. This is an obvious limitation for those with underlying chronic kidney disease particularly Stage 3 and above as it is potentially nephrotoxic. MRCA on the other hand utilizes the natural signal differences seen in SSFP imaging to visualize coronaries and does not require gadolinium contrast although it can be utilized. Currently used gadolinium compounds remain intravascular only for a short period of time thus limiting the benefit of contrast enhancement for MRCA for a short period of time. However some advances in MRI contrast agents have been made with newer agents with more prolonged intravascular time now being available. These agents increase contrast to noise ratio with MRCA and hold promise to improve diagnostic accuracy although no large scale studies have been performed as yet. It is important o note that gadolinium chelates can cause nephrogenic systemic fibrosis and are usually contraindicated in patients with glomerular filtration rates of < 30 ml/min.

19. Plaque imaging: CCTA versus MRCA

Plaque imaging is an exciting area of intense research and potential application of CCTA given its capacity to image the vessel wall and provide information beyond luminal narrowing. It can detect and characterize atherosclerotic plaques as calcified, non-calcified and mixed composition (Figure 10).[90] It is now known that regardless of degree of luminal stenosis even non-obstructive plaques as detected by CCTA carries adverse prognosis [91]. However, inter-observer variability of measurement of plaque dimensions is substantial and routine plaque measurements is not feasible at this time. However CCTA shows promise in identifying certain high risk characteristics such as bulky plaques, spotty calcification and positive remodeling all of which have been shown to be related to acute coronary syndromes [92]. With MRI, although once felt to be not possible, several investigators have imaged the coronary vessel wall and plaque successfully including subclinical wall thickening [93, 94], although from point of practical applicability this has yet to find a place in the clinical arena. Because of the lack of radiation exposure in MRCA it is ideally suited for follow-up imaging for assessing plaque progression [95] or to follow-up intermediate range stenosis where anatomy can be combined with a functional assessment of significance of lesion with stress –rest perfusion sequences [96].

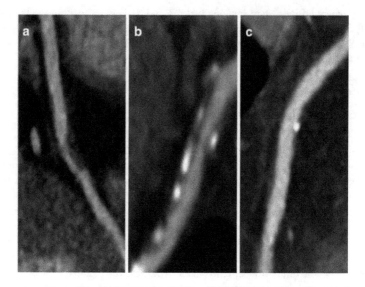

Figure 10.

20. Patient acceptance of CCTA versus MRCA

CCTA enjoys a much shorter time to completion of study compared to MRCA (20 versus 60 minutes respectively) which is a major attraction from the patient perspective [97]. For a modality to be overall successful in clinical practice it should not only be accurate, demonstrate clinical benefit and cost effective but also preferred by patients [98]. Studies have shown that patients prefer CCTA to MRCA [99]. This is mainly driven by longer imaging times, confinement in closed space and noise associated with MR imaging.

21. Training issues CCTA versus MRCA

Guidelines exist both from American College of Radiology [100] and the American College of Cardiology [101] for specific training requirements for gaining expertise in CCTA. Unfortunately no such guidelines exist for MRCA and given the complexity involved in image acquisition the degree of expertise needed to independently perform and interpret MRCA is likely to substantially greater with regards to training requirements. CCTA program clearly is easier to establish and execute than a MRCA program.

Table 5 summarizes various advantages and disadvantages from the authors perspective of CCTA and MRCA.

Properties	CTA	MRI
Time and patient preference	short duration and preffered	long duration, many breath holds, more claustrophobic
Comprehensive assessment	YES with higher radiation exposure, viability still not widely validated	one stop shop complete function, perfusion, viability and ischemic, myopathic assessment
Resolution	Higher spatial resolution	better temporal resolution
Diagnostic issues	superb negative predictive value and moderate positive predictive value	very good prognostic value in limited studies. Diagnostic values close to CT with 32C/3T
Radiation	yes	no
Calcification	interferes with interpretation	cannot be assessed. not limitation to assess coronaries
Radiocontrast	yes	no
Mettalic interference	yes but not contraindicated	currently contraindicated in pacemakers, defibrillators, metallic implants, shrapnel intracranial clips
Bypass Grafts	Excellent	Limited by artifacts
Stents	Large stents good	not good ?
Experience	Widespread	Limited
Availability	Widespread	Limited
Scanner	16Slice and Higher	1.5 T reasonable 3T better
Claustrophobia	Not a big issue	It is an issue
Irregular rhythm	Problem	Problem
Need premedication	Yes (mostly)	Not needed

Table 6.

22. Future perspectives

Noninvasive coronary angiography involving CCTA and MRCA has revolutionized delineation of coronary anatomy in a safe and fast way. CCTA has advanced much more in this aspect with fast imaging with single breath holds and 1 beat acquisition lasting a few seconds. The radiation and iodine based contrast are the major disadvantages although currently radiation doses below 1 millisievert are achievable with CCTA. MRCA with whole heart 3D imaging and 32 channel coils and 3T magnets have improved coronary imaging significantly but still lags behind and is not available widely. We foresee that CCTA will become mainstream for coronary imaging in low to intermediate risk populations with chest pains syndromes in the near future with exciting prospects of comprehensive cardiac imaging of perfusion and viability and plaque imaging.

Acknowledgements

We are indebted for the expert manuscript preparation assistance of Mrs Nandita S. Mani, MLIS, Sladen Library, Henry Ford Hospital, Detroit MI, USA

Author details

Karthikeyan Ananthasubramaniam[1*], Sabha Bhatti[1] and Abdul Hakeem[2]

*Address all correspondence to: kananth1@hfhs.org

1 Henry Ford Hospital, Heart and Vascular Institute, Detroit MI, USA

2 William Beaumont Hospital Royal Oak MI, USA

References

[1] Stuber M, Weiss RG. Coronary magnetic resonance angiography. Journal of magnetic resonance imaging: JMRI. 2007;26(2):219-34. Epub 2007/07/05.

[2] Manning WJ, Nezafat R, Appelbaum E, Danias PG, Hauser TH, Yeon SB. Coronary magnetic resonance imaging. Magnetic resonance imaging clinics of North America. 2007;15(4):609-37, vii. Epub 2007/11/03.

[3] Jahnke C, Paetsch I, Nehrke K, Schnackenburg B, Gebker R, Fleck E, et al. Rapid and complete coronary arterial tree visualization with magnetic resonance imaging: feasibility and diagnostic performance. European heart journal. 2005;26(21):2313-9. Epub 2005/07/01.

[4] Sakuma H, Ichikawa Y, Suzawa N, Hirano T, Makino K, Koyama N, et al. Assessment of coronary arteries with total study time of less than 30 minutes by using whole-heart coronary MR angiography. Radiology. 2005;237(1):316-21. Epub 2005/08/30.

[5] Nehrke K, Bornert P, Mazurkewitz P, Winkelmann R, Grasslin I. Free-breathing whole-heart coronary MR angiography on a clinical scanner in four minutes. Journal of magnetic resonance imaging : JMRI. 2006;23(5):752-6. Epub 2006/03/25.

[6] Wansapura J, Fleck R, Crotty E, Gottliebson W. Frequency scouting for cardiac imaging with SSFP at 3 Tesla. Pediatric radiology. 2006;36(10):1082-5. Epub 2006/07/11.

[7] Wang Y, Riederer SJ, Ehman RL. Respiratory motion of the heart: kinematics and the implications for the spatial resolution in coronary imaging. Magnetic resonance in

medicine : official journal of the Society of Magnetic Resonance in Medicine / Society of Magnetic Resonance in Medicine. 1995;33(5):713-9. Epub 1995/05/01.

[8]   Botnar RM, Stuber M, Danias PG, Kissinger KV, Manning WJ. Improved coronary artery definition with T2-weighted, free-breathing, three-dimensional coronary MRA. Circulation. 1999;99(24):3139-48. Epub 1999/06/22.

[9]   Jahnke C, Paetsch I, Achenbach S, Schnackenburg B, Gebker R, Fleck E, et al. Coronary MR imaging: breath-hold capability and patterns, coronary artery rest periods, and beta-blocker use. Radiology. 2006;239(1):71-8. Epub 2006/02/24.

[10] Ehman RL, Felmlee JP. Adaptive technique for high-definition MR imaging of moving structures. Radiology. 1989;173(1):255-63. Epub 1989/10/01.

[11] Johansson LO, Nolan MM, Taniuchi M, Fischer SE, Wickline SA, Lorenz CH. High-resolution magnetic resonance coronary angiography of the entire heart using a new blood-pool agent, NC100150 injection: comparison with invasive x-ray angiography in pigs. Journal of cardiovascular magnetic resonance : official journal of the Society for Cardiovascular Magnetic Resonance. 1999;1(2):139-43. Epub 2001/09/12.

[12] Li D, Dolan RP, Walovitch RC, Lauffer RB. Three-dimensional MRI of coronary arteries using an intravascular contrast agent. Magnetic resonance in medicine : official journal of the Society of Magnetic Resonance in Medicine / Society of Magnetic Resonance in Medicine. 1998;39(6):1014-8. Epub 1998/06/11.

[13] Snyder CJ, DelaBarre L, Metzger GJ, van de Moortele PF, Akgun C, Ugurbil K, et al. Initial results of cardiac imaging at 7 Tesla. Magnetic resonance in medicine : official journal of the Society of Magnetic Resonance in Medicine / Society of Magnetic Resonance in Medicine. 2009;61(3):517-24. Epub 2008/12/20.

[14] Bunce NH, Lorenz CH, Keegan J, Lesser J, Reyes EM, Firmin DN, et al. Coronary artery anomalies: assessment with free-breathing three-dimensional coronary MR angiography. Radiology. 2003;227(1):201-8. Epub 2003/02/26.

[15] Gharib AM, Ho VB, Rosing DR, Herzka DA, Stuber M, Arai AE, et al. Coronary artery anomalies and variants: technical feasibility of assessment with coronary MR angiography at 3 T. Radiology. 2008;247(1):220-7. Epub 2008/03/29.

[16] McConnell MV, Ganz P, Selwyn AP, Li W, Edelman RR, Manning WJ. Identification of anomalous coronary arteries and their anatomic course by magnetic resonance coronary angiography. Circulation. 1995;92(11):3158-62. Epub 1995/12/01.

[17] Post JC, van Rossum AC, Bronzwaer JG, de Cock CC, Hofman MB, Valk J, et al. Magnetic resonance angiography of anomalous coronary arteries. A new gold standard for delineating the proximal course? Circulation. 1995;92(11):3163-71. Epub 1995/12/01.

[18] Taylor AM, Thorne SA, Rubens MB, Jhooti P, Keegan J, Gatehouse PD, et al. Coronary artery imaging in grown up congenital heart disease: complementary role of

magnetic resonance and x-ray coronary angiography. Circulation. 2000;101(14): 1670-8. Epub 2000/04/12.

[19] Vliegen HW, Doornbos J, de Roos A, Jukema JW, Bekedam MA, van der Wall EE. Value of fast gradient echo magnetic resonance angiography as an adjunct to coronary arteriography in detecting and confirming the course of clinically significant coronary artery anomalies. The American journal of cardiology. 1997;79(6):773-6. Epub 1997/03/15.

[20] Kim WY, Danias PG, Stuber M, Flamm SD, Plein S, Nagel E, et al. Coronary magnetic resonance angiography for the detection of coronary stenoses. The New England journal of medicine. 2001;345(26):1863-9. Epub 2002/01/05.

[21] Sakuma H, Ichikawa Y, Chino S, Hirano T, Makino K, Takeda K. Detection of coronary artery stenosis with whole-heart coronary magnetic resonance angiography. Journal of the American College of Cardiology. 2006;48(10):1946-50. Epub 2006/11/23.

[22] Halliburton S, Arbab-Zadeh A, Dey D, Einstein AJ, Gentry R, George RT, et al. State-of-the-art in CT hardware and scan modes for cardiovascular CT. Journal of cardiovascular computed tomography. 2012;6(3):154-63. Epub 2012/05/04.

[23] 1990 Recommendations of the International Commission on Radiological Protection. Annals of the ICRP. 1991;21(1-3):1-201. Epub 1991/01/01.

[24] Alkadhi H, Stolzmann P, Scheffel H, Desbiolles L, Baumuller S, Plass A, et al. Radiation dose of cardiac dual-source CT: the effect of tailoring the protocol to patient-specific parameters. European journal of radiology. 2008;68(3):385-91. Epub 2008/11/04.

[25] Lell M, Marwan M, Schepis T, Pflederer T, Anders K, Flohr T, et al. Prospectively ECG-triggered high-pitch spiral acquisition for coronary CT angiography using dual source CT: technique and initial experience. European radiology. 2009;19(11):2576-83. Epub 2009/09/18.

[26] Gallagher MJ, Ross MA, Raff GL, Goldstein JA, O'Neill WW, O'Neil B. The diagnostic accuracy of 64-slice computed tomography coronary angiography compared with stress nuclear imaging in emergency department low-risk chest pain patients. Annals of emergency medicine. 2007;49(2):125-36. Epub 2006/09/19.

[27] Goldstein JA, Gallagher MJ, O'Neill WW, Ross MA, O'Neil BJ, Raff GL. A randomized controlled trial of multi-slice coronary computed tomography for evaluation of acute chest pain. Journal of the American College of Cardiology. 2007;49(8):863-71. Epub 2007/02/27.

[28] Hoffmann U, Bamberg F, Chae CU, Nichols JH, Rogers IS, Seneviratne SK, et al. Coronary computed tomography angiography for early triage of patients with acute chest pain: the ROMICAT (Rule Out Myocardial Infarction using Computer Assisted Tomography) trial. Journal of the American College of Cardiology. 2009;53(18): 1642-50. Epub 2009/05/02.

[29] Hollander JE, Chang AM, Shofer FS, McCusker CM, Baxt WG, Litt HI. Coronary computed tomographic angiography for rapid discharge of low-risk patients with potential acute coronary syndromes. Annals of emergency medicine. 2009;53(3): 295-304. Epub 2008/11/11.

[30] Leber AW, Knez A, von Ziegler F, Becker A, Nikolaou K, Paul S, et al. Quantification of obstructive and nonobstructive coronary lesions by 64-slice computed tomography: a comparative study with quantitative coronary angiography and intravascular ultrasound. Journal of the American College of Cardiology. 2005;46(1):147-54. Epub 2005/07/05.

[31] Leschka S, Alkadhi H, Plass A, Desbiolles L, Grunenfelder J, Marincek B, et al. Accuracy of MSCT coronary angiography with 64-slice technology: first experience. European heart journal. 2005;26(15):1482-7. Epub 2005/04/21.

[32] Pugliese F, Mollet NR, Hunink MG, Cademartiri F, Nieman K, van Domburg RT, et al. Diagnostic performance of coronary CT angiography by using different generations of multisection scanners: single-center experience. Radiology. 2008;246(2): 384-93. Epub 2008/01/09.

[33] Raff GL, Gallagher MJ, O'Neill WW, Goldstein JA. Diagnostic accuracy of noninvasive coronary angiography using 64-slice spiral computed tomography. Journal of the American College of Cardiology. 2005;46(3):552-7. Epub 2005/08/02.

[34] Rubinshtein R, Halon DA, Gaspar T, Jaffe R, Karkabi B, Flugelman MY, et al. Usefulness of 64-slice cardiac computed tomographic angiography for diagnosing acute coronary syndromes and predicting clinical outcome in emergency department patients with chest pain of uncertain origin. Circulation. 2007;115(13):1762-8. Epub 2007/03/21.

[35] Bluemke DA, Achenbach S, Budoff M, Gerber TC, Gersh B, Hillis LD, et al. Noninvasive coronary artery imaging: magnetic resonance angiography and multidetector computed tomography angiography: a scientific statement from the american heart association committee on cardiovascular imaging and intervention of the council on cardiovascular radiology and intervention, and the councils on clinical cardiology and cardiovascular disease in the young. Circulation. 2008;118(5):586-606. Epub 2008/07/01.

[36] Meijboom WB, Meijs MF, Schuijf JD, Cramer MJ, Mollet NR, van Mieghem CA, et al. Diagnostic accuracy of 64-slice computed tomography coronary angiography: a prospective, multicenter, multivendor study. Journal of the American College of Cardiology. 2008;52(25):2135-44. Epub 2008/12/20.

[37] Miller JM, Rochitte CE, Dewey M, Arbab-Zadeh A, Niinuma H, Gottlieb I, et al. Diagnostic performance of coronary angiography by 64-row CT. The New England journal of medicine. 2008;359(22):2324-36. Epub 2008/11/29.

[38] Chang SM, Bhatti S, Nabi F. Coronary computed tomography angiography. Current opinion in cardiology. 2011;26(5):392-402. Epub 2011/07/12.

[39] Cademartiri F, Maffei E, Palumbo A, Carrabba N, Ardissino D, Mollet N, et al. Multi-slice CT coronary angiography for the detection of in-stent restenosis. Current Cardiovascular Imaging Reports. 2008;1(2):119-24.

[40] Lu M, Jen-Sho Chen J, Awan O, White CS. Evaluation of Bypass Grafts and Stents. Radiologic clinics of North America. 2010;48(4):757-70.

[41] Gallagher MJ, Raff GL. Use of multislice CT for the evaluation of emergency room patients with chest pain: the so-called "triple rule-out". Catheterization and cardiovascular interventions : official journal of the Society for Cardiac Angiography & Interventions. 2008;71(1):92-9. Epub 2007/12/22.

[42] Gruettner J, Fink C, Walter T, Meyer M, Apfaltrer P, Schoepf UJ, et al. Coronary computed tomography and triple rule out CT in patients with acute chest pain and an intermediate cardiac risk profile. Part 1: Impact on patient management. European journal of radiology. 2012. Epub 2012/07/04.

[43] Samad Z, Hakeem A, Mahmood SS, Pieper K, Patel MR, Simel DL, et al. A meta-analysis and systematic review of computed tomography angiography as a diagnostic triage tool for patients with chest pain presenting to the emergency department. Journal of nuclear cardiology : official publication of the American Society of Nuclear Cardiology. 2012;19(2):364-76. Epub 2012/02/11.

[44] Litt HI, Gatsonis C, Snyder B, Singh H, Miller CD, Entrikin DW, et al. CT angiography for safe discharge of patients with possible acute coronary syndromes. The New England journal of medicine. 2012;366(15):1393-403. Epub 2012/03/28.

[45] Hoffmann U, Truong QA, Schoenfeld DA, Chou ET, Woodard PK, Nagurney JT, et al. Coronary CT angiography versus standard evaluation in acute chest pain. The New England journal of medicine. 2012;367(4):299-308. Epub 2012/07/27.

[46] Felker GM, Shaw LK, O'Connor CM. A standardized definition of ischemic cardiomyopathy for use in clinical research. Journal of the American College of Cardiology. 2002;39(2):210-8. Epub 2002/01/15.

[47] Bhatti S, Hakeem A, Yousuf MA, Al-Khalidi HR, Mazur W, Shizukuda Y. Diagnostic performance of computed tomography angiography for differentiating ischemic vs nonischemic cardiomyopathy. Journal of nuclear cardiology : official publication of the American Society of Nuclear Cardiology. 2011;18(3):407-20. Epub 2011/02/18.

[48] Moshage WE, Achenbach S, Seese B, Bachmann K, Kirchgeorg M. Coronary artery stenoses: three-dimensional imaging with electrocardiographically triggered, contrast agent-enhanced, electron-beam CT. Radiology. 1995;196(3):707-14. Epub 1995/09/01.

[49] Schuetz GM, Zacharopoulou NM, Schlattmann P, Dewey M. Meta-analysis: noninvasive coronary angiography using computed tomography versus magnetic resonance imaging. Annals of internal medicine. 2010;152(3):167-77. Epub 2010/02/04.

[50] Arbab-Zadeh A, Miller JM, Rochitte CE, Dewey M, Niinuma H, Gottlieb I, et al. Diagnostic accuracy of computed tomography coronary angiography according to pretest probability of coronary artery disease and severity of coronary arterial calcification. The CORE-64 (Coronary Artery Evaluation Using 64-Row Multidetector Computed Tomography Angiography) International Multicenter Study. Journal of the American College of Cardiology. 2012;59(4):379-87. Epub 2012/01/21.

[51] Hulten EA, Carbonaro S, Petrillo SP, Mitchell JD, Villines TC. Prognostic value of cardiac computed tomography angiography: a systematic review and meta-analysis. Journal of the American College of Cardiology. 2011;57(10):1237-47. Epub 2010/12/15.

[52] Bax JJ, Poldermans D, Schuijf JD, Scholte AJ, Elhendy A, van der Wall EE. Imaging to differentiate between ischemic and nonischemic cardiomyopathy. Heart failure clinics. 2006;2(2):205-14. Epub 2007/03/28.

[53] Dilsizian V, Pohost GM. Cardiac CT, PET, and MR. 2nd ed. Chichester, West Sussex, UK ; Hoboken, NJ: Wiley-Blackwell; 2010. ix, 374 p. p.

[54] Mark DB, Berman DS, Budoff MJ, Carr JJ, Gerber TC, Hecht HS, et al. ACCF/ACR/AHA/NASCI/SAIP/SCAI/SCCT 2010 expert consensus document on coronary computed tomographic angiography: a report of the American College of Cardiology Foundation Task Force on Expert Consensus Documents. Catheterization and cardiovascular interventions : official journal of the Society for Cardiac Angiography & Interventions. 2010;76(2):E1-42. Epub 2010/08/06.

[55] Meijboom WB, Van Mieghem CA, van Pelt N, Weustink A, Pugliese F, Mollet NR, et al. Comprehensive assessment of coronary artery stenoses: computed tomography coronary angiography versus conventional coronary angiography and correlation with fractional flow reserve in patients with stable angina. Journal of the American College of Cardiology. 2008;52(8):636-43. Epub 2008/08/16.

[56] Koo BK, Erglis A, Doh JH, Daniels DV, Jegere S, Kim HS, et al. Diagnosis of ischemia-causing coronary stenoses by noninvasive fractional flow reserve computed from coronary computed tomographic angiograms. Results from the prospective multicenter DISCOVER-FLOW (Diagnosis of Ischemia-Causing Stenoses Obtained Via Noninvasive Fractional Flow Reserve) study. Journal of the American College of Cardiology. 2011;58(19):1989-97. Epub 2011/10/29.

[57] Hoe J. CT coronary angiography of chronic total occlusions of the coronary arteries: how to recognize and evaluate and usefulness for planning percutaneous coronary interventions. The international journal of cardiovascular imaging. 2009;25 Suppl 1:43-54. Epub 2009/01/24.

[58] Carrabba N, Schuijf JD, de Graaf FR, Parodi G, Maffei E, Valenti R, et al. Diagnostic accuracy of 64-slice computed tomography coronary angiography for the detection of in-stent restenosis: a meta-analysis. Journal of nuclear cardiology : official publication of the American Society of Nuclear Cardiology. 2010;17(3):470-8. Epub 2010/04/10.

[59] Flohr TG, Raupach R, Bruder H. Cardiac CT: how much can temporal resolution, spatial resolution, and volume coverage be improved? Journal of cardiovascular computed tomography. 2009;3(3):143-52. Epub 2009/06/17.

[60] Einstein AJ, Moser KW, Thompson RC, Cerqueira MD, Henzlova MJ. Radiation dose to patients from cardiac diagnostic imaging. Circulation. 2007;116(11):1290-305. Epub 2007/09/12.

[61] Gerber TC, Carr JJ, Arai AE, Dixon RL, Ferrari VA, Gomes AS, et al. Ionizing radiation in cardiac imaging: a science advisory from the American Heart Association Committee on Cardiac Imaging of the Council on Clinical Cardiology and Committee on Cardiovascular Imaging and Intervention of the Council on Cardiovascular Radiology and Intervention. Circulation. 2009;119(7):1056-65. Epub 2009/02/04.

[62] Higgins CB, Siemers PT, Newell JD, Schmidt W. Role of iodinated contrast material in the evaluation of myocardial infarction by computerized transmission tomography. Investigative radiology. 1980;15(6 Suppl):S176-82. Epub 1980/11/01.

[63] Mahnken AH, Koos R, Katoh M, Wildberger JE, Spuentrup E, Buecker A, et al. Assessment of myocardial viability in reperfused acute myocardial infarction using 16-slice computed tomography in comparison to magnetic resonance imaging. Journal of the American College of Cardiology. 2005;45(12):2042-7. Epub 2005/06/21.

[64] George RT, Arbab-Zadeh A, Miller JM, Kitagawa K, Chang HJ, Bluemke DA, et al. Adenosine stress 64- and 256-row detector computed tomography angiography and perfusion imaging: a pilot study evaluating the transmural extent of perfusion abnormalities to predict atherosclerosis causing myocardial ischemia. Circulation Cardiovascular imaging. 2009;2(3):174-82. Epub 2009/10/08.

[65] Rumberger JA, Feiring AJ, Lipton MJ, Higgins CB, Ell SR, Marcus ML. Use of ultrafast computed tomography to quantitate regional myocardial perfusion: a preliminary report. Journal of the American College of Cardiology. 1987;9(1):59-69. Epub 1987/01/01.

[66] Williams MC, Reid JH, McKillop G, Weir NW, van Beek EJ, Uren NG, et al. Cardiac and coronary CT comprehensive imaging approach in the assessment of coronary heart disease. Heart. 2011;97(15):1198-205. Epub 2011/07/12.

[67] Foo TK, Ho VB, Saranathan M, Cheng LQ, Sakuma H, Kraitchman DL, et al. Feasibility of integrating high-spatial-resolution 3D breath-hold coronary MR angiography with myocardial perfusion and viability examinations. Radiology. 2005;235(3):1025-30. Epub 2005/05/26.

[68] Plein S, Jones TR, Ridgway JP, Sivananthan MU. Three-dimensional coronary MR angiography performed with subject-specific cardiac acquisition windows and motion-adapted respiratory gating. AJR American journal of roentgenology. 2003;180(2):505-12. Epub 2003/01/24.

[69] Dewey M. Coronary CT versus MR angiography: pro CT--the role of CT angiography. Radiology. 2011;258(2):329-39. Epub 2011/01/29.

[70] Hamdan A, Asbach P, Wellnhofer E, Klein C, Gebker R, Kelle S, et al. A prospective study for comparison of MR and CT imaging for detection of coronary artery stenosis. JACC Cardiovascular imaging. 2011;4(1):50-61. Epub 2011/01/15.

[71] Hendel RC, Patel MR, Kramer CM, Poon M, Hendel RC, Carr JC, et al. ACCF/ACR/ SCCT/SCMR/ASNC/NASCI/SCAI/SIR 2006 appropriateness criteria for cardiac computed tomography and cardiac magnetic resonance imaging: a report of the American College of Cardiology Foundation Quality Strategic Directions Committee Appropriateness Criteria Working Group, American College of Radiology, Society of Cardiovascular Computed Tomography, Society for Cardiovascular Magnetic Resonance, American Society of Nuclear Cardiology, North American Society for Cardiac Imaging, Society for Cardiovascular Angiography and Interventions, and Society of Interventional Radiology. Journal of the American College of Cardiology. 2006;48(7): 1475-97. Epub 2006/10/03.

[72] Kleinerman RA. Cancer risks following diagnostic and therapeutic radiation exposure in children. Pediatric radiology. 2006;36 Suppl 2:121-5. Epub 2006/07/25.

[73] McCarthy RM, Shea SM, Deshpande VS, Green JD, Pereles FS, Carr JC, et al. Coronary MR angiography: true FISP imaging improved by prolonging breath holds with preoxygenation in healthy volunteers. Radiology. 2003;227(1):283-8. Epub 2003/03/05.

[74] Liu X, Bi X, Huang J, Jerecic R, Carr J, Li D. Contrast-enhanced whole-heart coronary magnetic resonance angiography at 3.0 T: comparison with steady-state free precession technique at 1.5 T. Investigative radiology. 2008;43(9):663-8. Epub 2008/08/19.

[75] Yang Q, Li K, Liu X, Bi X, Liu Z, An J, et al. Contrast-enhanced whole-heart coronary magnetic resonance angiography at 3.0-T: a comparative study with X-ray angiography in a single center. Journal of the American College of Cardiology. 2009;54(1): 69-76. Epub 2009/06/27.

[76] Greil GF, Stuber M, Botnar RM, Kissinger KV, Geva T, Newburger JW, et al. Coronary magnetic resonance angiography in adolescents and young adults with kawasaki disease. Circulation. 2002;105(8):908-11. Epub 2002/02/28.

[77] Mavrogeni S, Papadopoulos G, Douskou M, Kaklis S, Seimenis I, Baras P, et al. Magnetic resonance angiography is equivalent to X-ray coronary angiography for the evaluation of coronary arteries in Kawasaki disease. Journal of the American College of Cardiology. 2004;43(4):649-52. Epub 2004/02/21.

[78] Wang L, Jerosch-Herold M, Jacobs DR, Jr., Shahar E, Detrano R, Folsom AR, et al. Coronary artery calcification and myocardial perfusion in asymptomatic adults: the MESA (Multi-Ethnic Study of Atherosclerosis). Journal of the American College of Cardiology. 2006;48(5):1018-26. Epub 2006/09/05.

[79] Brodoefel H, Burgstahler C, Tsiflikas I, Reimann A, Schroeder S, Claussen CD, et al. Dual-source CT: effect of heart rate, heart rate variability, and calcification on image quality and diagnostic accuracy. Radiology. 2008;247(2):346-55. Epub 2008/03/29.

[80] Liu X, Zhao X, Huang J, Francois CJ, Tuite D, Bi X, et al. Comparison of 3D free-breathing coronary MR angiography and 64-MDCT angiography for detection of coronary stenosis in patients with high calcium scores. AJR American journal of roentgenology. 2007;189(6):1326-32. Epub 2007/11/22.

[81] McCarthy JH, Palmer FJ. Incidence and significance of coronary artery calcification. British heart journal. 1974;36(5):499-506. Epub 1974/05/01.

[82] Hecht HS, Budoff MJ, Berman DS, Ehrlich J, Rumberger JA. Coronary artery calcium scanning: Clinical paradigms for cardiac risk assessment and treatment. American heart journal. 2006;151(6):1139-46. Epub 2006/06/20.

[83] McLaughlin VV, Balogh T, Rich S. Utility of electron beam computed tomography to stratify patients presenting to the emergency room with chest pain. The American journal of cardiology. 1999;84(3):327-8, A8. Epub 1999/09/25.

[84] Greenland P, LaBree L, Azen SP, Doherty TM, Detrano RC. Coronary artery calcium score combined with Framingham score for risk prediction in asymptomatic individuals. JAMA : the journal of the American Medical Association. 2004;291(2):210-5. Epub 2004/01/15.

[85] Liu ZY, Gao CQ, Li BJ, Wu Y, Xiao CS, Ye WH, et al. [Diagnostic study on the coronary artery bypass grafts lesions using 64 multi-slice computed tomography angiography]. Zhonghua wai ke za zhi [Chinese journal of surgery]. 2008;46(4):245-7. Epub 2008/08/08.

[86] Langerak SE, Vliegen HW, de Roos A, Zwinderman AH, Jukema JW, Kunz P, et al. Detection of vein graft disease using high-resolution magnetic resonance angiography. Circulation. 2002;105(3):328-33. Epub 2002/01/24.

[87] Antoniucci D, Valenti R, Santoro GM, Bolognese L, Trapani M, Cerisano G, et al. Restenosis after coronary stenting in current clinical practice. American heart journal. 1998;135(3):510-8. Epub 1998/03/20.

[88] Hug J, Nagel E, Bornstedt A, Schnackenburg B, Oswald H, Fleck E. Coronary arterial stents: safety and artifacts during MR imaging. Radiology. 2000;216(3):781-7. Epub 2000/08/31.

[89] Maintz D, Botnar RM, Fischbach R, Heindel W, Manning WJ, Stuber M. Coronary magnetic resonance angiography for assessment of the stent lumen: a phantom study. Journal of cardiovascular magnetic resonance : official journal of the Society for Cardiovascular Magnetic Resonance. 2002;4(3):359-67. Epub 2002/09/18.

[90] Maurovich-Horvat P, Ferencik M, Bamberg F, Hoffmann U. Methods of plaque quantification and characterization by cardiac computed tomography. Journal of cardiovascular computed tomography. 2009;3 Suppl 2:S91-8. Epub 2010/02/05.

[91] Pundziute G, Schuijf JD, Jukema JW, Boersma E, de Roos A, van der Wall EE, et al. Prognostic value of multislice computed tomography coronary angiography in pa-

tients with known or suspected coronary artery disease. Journal of the American College of Cardiology. 2007;49(1):62-70. Epub 2007/01/09.

[92] Motoyama S, Sarai M, Harigaya H, Anno H, Inoue K, Hara T, et al. Computed tomographic angiography characteristics of atherosclerotic plaques subsequently resulting
in acute coronary syndrome. Journal of the American College of Cardiology.
2009;54(1):49-57. Epub 2009/06/27.

[93] Botnar RM, Stuber M, Lamerichs R, Smink J, Fischer SE, Harvey P, et al. Initial experiences with in vivo right coronary artery human MR vessel wall imaging at 3 tesla.
Journal of cardiovascular magnetic resonance : official journal of the Society for Cardiovascular Magnetic Resonance. 2003;5(4):589-94. Epub 2003/12/11.

[94] Fayad ZA, Fuster V, Fallon JT, Jayasundera T, Worthley SG, Helft G, et al. Noninvasive in vivo human coronary artery lumen and wall imaging using black-blood magnetic resonance imaging. Circulation. 2000;102(5):506-10. Epub 2000/08/02.

[95] Botnar RM, Stuber M, Kissinger KV, Kim WY, Spuentrup E, Manning WJ. Noninvasive coronary vessel wall and plaque imaging with magnetic resonance imaging. Circulation. 2000;102(21):2582-7. Epub 2000/11/22.

[96] Nikolaou K, Alkadhi H, Bamberg F, Leschka S, Wintersperger BJ. MRI and CT in the
diagnosis of coronary artery disease: indications and applications. Insights into imaging. 2011;2(1):9-24. Epub 2012/02/22.

[97] Dewey M, Teige F, Schnapauff D, Laule M, Borges AC, Wernecke KD, et al. Noninvasive detection of coronary artery stenoses with multislice computed tomography or
magnetic resonance imaging. Annals of internal medicine. 2006;145(6):407-15. Epub
2006/09/20.

[98] Genders TS, Meijboom WB, Meijs MF, Schuijf JD, Mollet NR, Weustink AC, et al. CT
coronary angiography in patients suspected of having coronary artery disease: decision making from various perspectives in the face of uncertainty. Radiology.
2009;253(3):734-44. Epub 2009/10/30.

[99] Schonenberger E, Schnapauff D, Teige F, Laule M, Hamm B, Dewey M. Patient acceptance of noninvasive and invasive coronary angiography. PloS one.
2007;2(2):e246. Epub 2007/03/01.

[100] Jacobs JE, Boxt LM, Desjardins B, Fishman EK, Larson PA, Schoepf J, et al. ACR practice guideline for the performance and interpretation of cardiac computed tomography (CT). Journal of the American College of Radiology : JACR. 2006;3(9):677-85.
Epub 2007/04/07.

[101] Budoff MJ, Cohen MC, Garcia MJ, Hodgson JM, Hundley WG, Lima JA, et al.
ACCF/AHA clinical competence statement on cardiac imaging with computed tomography and magnetic resonance: a report of the American College of Cardiology
Foundation/American Heart Association/American College of Physicians Task Force
on Clinical Competence and Training. Journal of the American College of Cardiology. 2005;46(2):383-402. Epub 2005/07/19.

Chapter 4

Radiation Principles and Safety

Jasmin Čaluk

Additional information is available at the end of the chapter

1. Introduction

Interventional cardiology today without the use of x-ray technology cannot even be imagined. This is also true for medicine in general. The radiology era begins with the discovery of the x-rays by Wilhelm Conrad Röntgen, on the November 8th 1895 (following the transliteration conventions for the characters accentuated by 'umlaut', „Röntgen" is in English spelled „Roentgen", and with that spelling is most often found in the literature). On that day he produced and detected for the first time the electromagnetic radiation in the wavelengths today known as the x-rays, for which he received the Nobel prize for physics in 1901 [1]. This was the start of radiology, which has developed tremendously over the years. In time, radiology adopted other forms of human body imaging (magnetic resonance, positron emission tomography etc.), but even today the most radiologic studies in the world are performed using the x-rays, whether in the form of classic x-ray imaging, computer tomography, or various forms of fluoroscopy and/or fluorography, which is used in interventional cardiology. The term 'fluoroscopy' depicts viewing of structures in real time, while 'fluorography' means that different methods of image aquisition and storage for later review are being used.

X-ray radiation is a form of electromagnetic radiation. X-rays are electromagnetic waves with a wavelength in the range of 0.01 to 10 nanometers, which corresponds to frequencies in the range 30 petahertz to 30 exahertz (3×10^{16} Hz to 3×10^{19} Hz) and energies in the range 120 eV to 120 keV. X-rays are shorter in wavelength than ultra-violet rays and longer than gamma rays. In many languages, X-radiation is called Röntgen radiation, after Wilhelm Conrad Röntgen, who is usually credited as its discoverer, and who had actually named it X-radiation to signify the up to then unknown type of radiation [1].

X-ray input doses for fluorography are generally 10-fold higher than those used for fluoroscopy. This is why fluorography is the major source of the radiation dose [2]. Procedures which include the use of x-rays are associated with the exposure of the patients to a certain amount of x-ray radiation, and in some cases, especially in interventional cardiology, the staff is also exposed to this form of radiation. The constant evolution of interventional cardiology, with ever more complex procedures demanding prolonged fluoroscopy and fluorography time, as well as the demands for better imaging of small structures (guidewires, angioplasty balloon- and stent-markers, stents themselves, intravascular ultrasound probes, etc.) associated with higher exposures to larger amounts of x-ray radiation, have all raised the question of radiation protection, both for the patients and the staff inside the catheterization laboratory (cath lab). Occupational doses of radiation in interventional cardiology procedures guided by fluoroscopy are the highest doses registered among medical staff using x-rays. The use of ionizing radiation increases the risk of malignant disease occurrence and can cause skin or eye damage to both the patient and the personnel [3].

2. How the x-ray radiation is produced

2.1. The x-ray tube

The principle of generating the x-rays is basically the same in all x-ray machines. The source of x-rays is the x-ray tube (fig.1, fig. 2). Within it are the cathode and the anode (fig. 1). The electrically positive tungsten anode is bombarded with accelerated electrons originating from the electrically negative cathode. When the high-velocity electrons collide with the anode, they lose most of their energy (~99%) as heat, and a small fraction (~1%) as x-rays. Since the electrons are slowed down within the anode by different segments of atoms and mostly multiple interactions with several atoms within the material itself, they release a variety of x-ray energies. However, when all of the electron's energy is lost in a single interaction, the resultant emitted x-ray has the highest possible energy, equivalent to the voltage applied across the tube. That is reffered to as the kVp, or 'peak kilovoltage' of the emitted x-rays. A typical x-ray tube ranges from 60 kV to 120 kV. The tube current, measured in milliamperes (mA) is defined as the number of electrons that arc from the cathode to the anode per second [4]. Modern x-ray tubes generate the radiation in pulses rather than in a continuous form, and those pulses are synchronized with the other components in the fluoroscopic/fluorographic system. The duration of the time during which the electrons hit the anode is the pulse width, and is measured in milliseconds (ms).

The anode is made of tungsten because this material can withstand very high temperatures without melting. As stated before, some 99% of the energy which the electron beam is losing when hitting the anode is heat. The anode is constructed as a disc, and to reduce the heat strain even more, it is constantly rotated at speeds up to 10,000 rpm (fig. 1). This way, the area bombarded by the small electron beam is not actually a single spot, but a circle track. The small area of the anode which is being bombarded by the electron beam, and from which the x-rays are emitted is called the 'focal spot', and since the anode is being rotated, the focal spot is actually the already described circular track on the anode disc. The size of the focal spot affects the image quality in different ways. If it is smaller, the images are sharper, but if it is larger, it can produce more x-rays. The cathode is a tungsten wire, and is the source of electrons which are accelerated towards the anode. The cathode is heated to high temperatures by passing the current through it, and is maintained at a large negative voltage relative to the anode. The electrons are 'fired away' from it and accelerate toward the anode, hitting it as they reach their maximum energy, which is 60 kV to 120 kV.

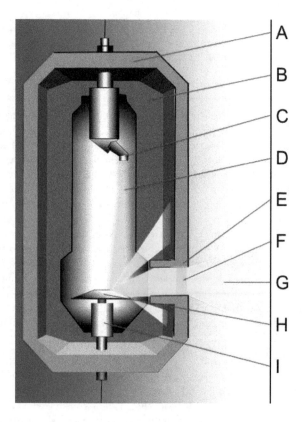

Figure 1. The x-ray tube. Legend: A – housing; B – oil bath for cooling; C – cathode; D – electron beam; E – collimators; F – filters; G – x-rays; H – anode; I – engine for anode rotation (illustration: J. Čaluk).

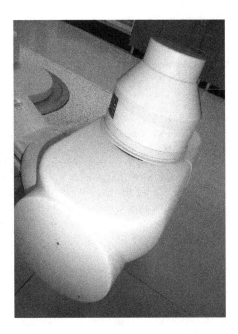

Figure 2. X-ray tube

2.2. Filters

As the electrons are slowed down by the anode, there occurs a spectrum of different wavelength x-rays called the brake-radiation (in German: Bremsstrahlung), with spikes of x-ray energies at characteristic wavelengths when all the energy of an electron is lost at a single collision, as noted earlier. The brake-radiation is mostly of low photon energies (<25-30 keV), and would be mostly absorbed in the patient's superfitial tissues. Therefore, the brake-radiation would not contribute to generating the x-ray image, but would, on the other hand, increase the amount of radiation to which the patient is exposed. This is why these x-rays are filtered in the beam exit port, and the filters applied selectively absorb the x-ray photons from this region of the energy spectrum [4]. Modern systems usually use copper filters 0.2 – 0.9 mm thick. Since these filters attenuate the x-ray beam (fig. 1), this requires an increased tube output, and when this is accomplished, the greater energy output occurs in the energy range of interest. Filters are basically simple, small metal sheets. In addition to the permanent beam filtration that is usually equivalent to 3 mm of aluminium, all cardio-angiographic equipment should have heavily filtered x-ray sources. The number and the mode of filter use differs among manufacturers, but optional filters of 0.1 mm, 0.2 mm, 0.3 mm, etc. should be available to order with the machine. In some products, users can employ different dose-management modes, and these filters might be incorporated into those modes, selectable by the user.

The thickest filters would therefore be used for smaller patients, and the thinnest ones for large patients. Since the filters primarily eliminate the useless part of the x-ray beam, but also do attenuate even a part of the useful beam, the goal of filtration is to produce the best possible compromise between image quality and radiation dose.

2.3. Collimators

In order to adjust the shape and the size of the x-ray field emerging from the tube, lead collimators which completely absorb the x-ray beam are used. They actually limit the exposure of the patient only within the region of interest, and thus reduce the unneccessary exposure to both the patient and the staff. The collimators can be manipulated as to further reduce the port of the x-ray tube (fig. 1) and by that, to reduce the irradiated area. The edges of the collimator blades are then visible in the imaging field as shadows. The amount of absorbed and scattered radiation can be reduced by an adequate collimation –the entrance surface area of the x-ray beam on the patient's skin should be reduced to the smallest possible/needed size [5,6,7].

2.4. X-ray generators

The x-ray generator provides the electric power to heat the cathode, to accelerate the electrons from the cathode to the anode thus generating the x-ray beam, and to turn the x-ray pulses on and off. It automatically adjusts the tube voltage, current, and pulse width to maintain a certain image quality. In interventional cardiology, there is a demand for generators able to provide up to 100 kW of power across all the voltages in the diagnostic range. The modulation of variables of x-ray beams is automated, and it maintains constant brightness at the image receptor as the thickness of patient's tissues varies with different projections and angulations. Very oblique angulations mean that the tissue thickness is bigger, and more powerful radiation is required to generate the image in comparison to less or non-angulated tube positions. Also, the image quality must be maintained regardless of the patient's built, so bigger patients are exposed to higher amounts of radiation, because stronger x-ray beams are required to penetrate their bodies [8,9]. Image brightness at the oputput of the imaging chain is rapidly sampled. The measurements are sent back to the generator to modulate the above mentioned variables and provide the desired image brightness. Beside the pulse width, the voltage, and the current, the parameters which can be altered are camera aperture and electronic amplification gain.

3. X-ray image formation

The x-ray beam directed towards the patient is considered to be uniform. After interacting with different tissues which attenuate it to a variable degree, a non-uniform x-ray beam exits the patient. Its non-uniformity, generated by the process of x-ray absorption in the patient, is the basis for obtaining an x-ray image. The degree of 'darkness' in the x-ray image, which forms the x-ray 'shadow', is determined by the energy of the original x-ray beam generated by the tube, the thickness of the exposed object (patient's tissues), and the elemental makeup of the object (patient's tissues). The removal of the x-ray beam as a function of the object thickness is exponential, but the elemental makeup of the tissue is characteristic for the tissue itself, and as a function is characterized by a linear attenuation coefficient. Half-value layer (HVL) is the parameter defined as the thickness of a tissue sample that absorbes (removes from the beam) one-half of the beam intensity. Regarding the beam energies used in interventional cardiology, HVL for muscle would be 3.2 cm, for bone is 1.5 cm, for iodine is 0.01 cm (100%), and as a comparison, for the lead, the HVL is 0.01 cm [4].

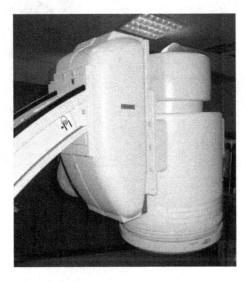

Figure 3. Image intensifier

When a non-uniform x-ray beam leaves the patient's body, its spatial distribution is the basis for forming an x-ray image. It contains the information on the anatomy of the scanned region, and if it is taken within a defined time-frame, it can also be used for the assessment of the patient's physiology. But, since the spectrum of x-rays cannot be detected by the human eyes, it must be 'translated' into visible information. There are several technologies currently in use for that purpose, and the most common being used in interventional cardiology today are image intensifier and digital flat-panel detector technology, both of which are digital. Although our senses use the analogue method to percieve the reality, for the purpose of securely storing the information and being possible to make exact copies, and later review the information without quality loss, that information needs to be digitalized. The digital-flat panel detectors are the state of the art now, but still the vast majority of the systems currently in use employ the image intensifier technology (fig. 3). The main role of the image intensifier is to convert the x-ray intensity information into the visible light spectrum and expose photographic film or a video camera. The details of the process taking place within the image intensifier are beyond the scope of this chapter and are discussed elsewhere.

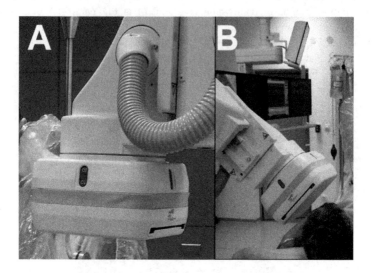

Figure 4. Digital flat-panel detector

However, recently a novel technology has been introduced and its use in cardio-angiography is constantly increasing: the digital flat-panel detector (fig. 4), which consists of (simply speaking) several layers of material. The x-ray photons, upon leaving the patient, hit the input phosphor layer of the detector, and it produces light photons. Behind that layer is the photodiode and the thin-film transistor layer. The generated light photons produce electric signals within this layer, and those signals are captured as voltages in the discrete flat-panel elements [4]. A typical panel consists of 1024 x 1024 elements over a rectangle-shaped field of view. Each flat-panel element's voltage signal is converted from an analogue voltage to a digital representation. The digital image produced like this is represented using a fixed number of values, and those are distributed over a limited set of co-ordinates. This information can then be stored or copied. For viewing, it is fed through conversion system and into the viewing monitor, and we percieve it as an image, with monitor pixels corresponding to flat panel detector's elements which received the beam. In order to standardize the digital communication within the medical community, the DICOM (Digital Imaging Communications in Medicine) system has been introduced. It is used for organizing the image data in such a way that other users of the DICOM system can review those data accurately, and is currently the standard-one in medicine.

4. Radiation management and safety

X-ray radiation is a carcinogen [10]. No dose of radiation may be considered safe or harmless [11]. It can also cause severe injury called radiation burns, but the likelihood of that is extremely low when the fluoroscopy/fluorography is adequately managed. Doctors, nurses, technicians, and other medical staff working in radiation environment, who have accumulated significant doses of radiation through their careers have been shown to develop some form of radiation-induced health-problems, the most important being cancer, cataracts, and skin injury [12,13]. Interventional cardiologists, working at very low distances from x-ray tubes, and the patients who are also the sources of scattered radiation, are at particular health risk.

4.1. Radiation effects

Effects of radiation can be generally divided into two basic groups: the stochastic effects, and the deterministic effects. Both groups are very important for the pathological consequences on the human body.

Stochastic effect occurs within a single cell and makes it adversely functional. This happens because of an alteration of an important macromolecule (such as the DNA) and can result upon a single interaction with radiation. It is therefore logical to assume that this kind of effects may occur with any radiation dose, but in practice, low doses of radiation carry an extremely low risk of stochastic effects on the body. The most important stochastic effects in the clinical sense are the occurrence of radiation-induced tumors and heritable changes in reproductive cells. The risk of these effects occurring rises with the rise of the amount of radiation to which a person is exposed, so the induced cancer becomes measurable in exposed adults at doses over some 100 mSv. In children, and in fetus (if a pregnant woman is exposed to radiation), even lower doses have been defined as carcinogenic. The stochastic risk of inducing malignant disease associated with radiation is small but definite [14].

Deterministic effects are the result of damage to a large number of cells, therefore a certain dose of radiation has to be applied for these effects to take place. This minimal dose for a deterministic effect is called the threshold dose. The higher the dose (above the threshold), the more severe the effects. Some examples of deterministic effects are: skin erythema, epilation, dry or moist desquamation, secondary ulceration, ischemic dermal necrosis, various stages of dermal atrophy, induration, teleangiectasia, late dermal necrosis, vision-impairing cataract [10]. Some authors propose that skin cancer can also be considered to be a deterministic effect of radiation.

For both of these groups of radiation effects there exists a time delay between the exposure to radiation and the clinical manifestation of the effect itself. This delay ranges from days to weeks to months for deterministic effects, and for malignant diseases, from as little as 2 years, to as long as many decades. In many cases, neither the patient, nor the physician (usually a dermatologists or a general practitioner) grasps the connection of a skin disorder (usually an erythema, or a 'radiation burn') and a previous interventional cardiology procedure, because of this time delay – usually several weeks.

4.2. Units of measurement of x-ray radiation

In order to understand and quantify the effects of radiation on humans, different units of measurement have been developed. It is necessary to know these units as to be able to apply the safety measures in radiation environment, as well as to compare the health-risks of different forms of radiation.

Absorbed dose is the amount of radiation energy absorbed by a particular tissue. The x-ray radiation interacts with living tissues upon entering them, and its energy causes molecular changes, and therefore has the potential to have biologic effects. The unit of absorbed dose is gray (Gy), meaning that 1 Gy is the radiation energy of one joule (1 J) concentrated in one kilogram (1 kg) of tissue.

Equivalent dose is an estimate of the biologic potency which a form of radiation might have for an absorbed dose, and is determined by the properties of the radiation itself. Therefore, for different kinds of radiation, the equivalent doses can be different, although the absorbed doses can be the same. This is actually a safety term that can be used to compare the biologic potency of different kinds of radiation. The unit for equivalent dose is sievert (Sv). In interventional cardiology, 1 Sv is considered to be equivalent to 1 Gy [10].

Effective dose is the estimate of a hypothetic dose which would have to be delivered to an interventionist's entire body to have the same risk for the radiation adverse effects as the non-uniform doses which are actually delivered. The need for establishing this unit of measurement occurred because during the procedures in the cath lab (or similar radiation environments), some of the body parts are better protected (e.g. internal organs), while other body parts are less, or not at all protected (e.g. head and limbs), under the assumption that they are less radiosensitive. Therefore, the spatial distribution of radiation exposure is non-uniform. Effective dose eliminates this complexity in radiation risk assessment. The unit to measure the effective dose is sievert (Sv), and in interventional cardiology 1 Sv can be considered to be equal to 1 Gy of x-ray radiation absorbed uniformly in the body.

There are, of course, the proposed limits to which personnel in the radiation environment can be exposed. Regarding the effective dose, the limit for the staff is 100 mSv in a consecutive five year period, subject to a maximum effective dose of 50 mSv in any single year. The equivalent dose for the lenses of the eye should be limited to 150 mSv in a year. The limit on equivalent dose for the skin should be 500 mSv in a year, and the dose for the hands, forearms, feet, and ankles should be limited to 500 mSv in a year [11].

4.3. Limiting the exposure to radiation

The basic rule which can be applied regarding radiation protection is: 'what is good for the patient is also good for the staff'. For this reason, radiation protection measures will be discussed in general, with additional comments regarding the staff or the patient when necessary. The four basic methods of limiting exposure to radiation can be remembered by using the mnemonic TIDS, which stands for: time, intensity, distance, and shielding [10].

The time of fluoroscopy/fluorography should be limited to the necessary minimum. A good measure for orientation regarding this is fluoroscopy time recorded by most machines used for cardio-angiography today. Although, most devices show only fluoroscopy time, and the operator must also think about the fluorography time, knowing that the amount of radiation for the same amount of time is in fluorography 10-fold of that in fluoroscopy. Some devices have the ability to show fluorography time, or a complete beam-on time. In addition, a trend towards less fluoroscopy time is obvious with more experienced operators. However, more experienced operators are more often involved in complex procedures, which actually prolong the fluoroscopy time. Regardless of that, all operators have to be aware that they must reduce the beam-on time to a minimum provided that they can visualize the structures of interest and complete the procedure safely. Complex procedures, such as multivessel interventions, treating chronic total occlusions, or bifurcation lesions demand more procedure time than the simple interventions, and this leads to increased radiation dose when treating more complex coronary disease [16]. Some practical advices: when documenting balloon inflation, just a short single shot should be enough, there is no need to prolong the shot of an inflated balloon; there is no reason to record or observe the gradual balloon deflation, this can be checked with short beam-on shots; the operator's foot should be kept away from the fluoropedal when not actually using fluorography, as to not accidentally step on the pedal and produce unnecessary radiation; a diagnostic fluorography can in most cases (but not always) be limited to a single cardiac cyclus; direct stenting can also be used and is proven to reduce beam-on time [17,18].

Intensity of radiation should also be minimized. This can be done in several ways. As noted earlier, the tube current and voltage can be modulated up to a point. An easier way to reduce the intensity would be by reducing the pulse rate, in some devices marked as 'frame rate'. This can also be done to a point where the radiation is minimal, while the images are adequate for performing the procedure.

Distance from the source of radiation must be maximized. It is advisable for the operator to stand away from the tube as much as possible, while being able to operate the equipment, the catheters, syringes, etc. Regarding the other staff in the cath lab, anyone who is not needed inside the room should leave the room, but be readily available to enter as soon as they are needed. All the members of the staff who must stay inside the cath lab should keep their distance from the radiation source at all times, but be ready to attend the patient, or assist the operator on demand. Even small increase of distance from the source of radiation is important, because for each doubling of distance from the source, the intensity of radiation is reduced 4-fold.

Shielding of personnel from the radiation is also of utmost importance. The radiation shields come in several types. The ones above the patient are connected to an anchor point in the ceiling and should be moveable, so that they can be adjusted to the patient's position and size (fig. 5, fig. 6). These shields protect the operator and the assisting staff from the radiation scattered from the patient's body. Some cardio-angiographic tables have the lower shields attached at the table sides, and the angulation of those shields can be altered to provide the best possible operator and staff protection from the scattered radiation off the posterior aspect of the supine patient, but also from the radiation generated by the tube, which is located beneath the patient (fig. 5, fig. 6). These shielding drapes significantly protect the operator from scattered radiation [19,20]. In some cases these shields are not connected to the tables themselves, but are free-standing. These shields protect the operator's legs and feet, which are among the most exposed body parts of the operator. There is further shielding in the walls, floors, and the ceiling of the cath lab in order to protect the people outside the cath lab.

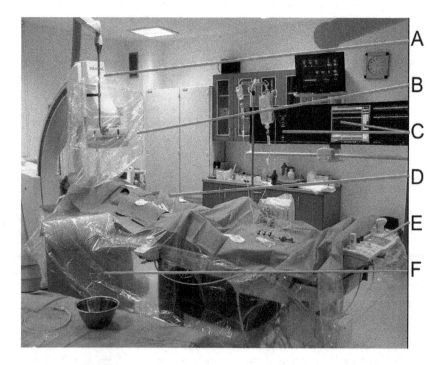

Figure 5. Patient position and shielding in the cath lab. Legend: A – digital flat panel detector mounted on C-arm; B – ceiling-mounted articulated protection screen; C – monitors; D – patient; E – C-arm and image contriol panel; F – table-side protective shielding.

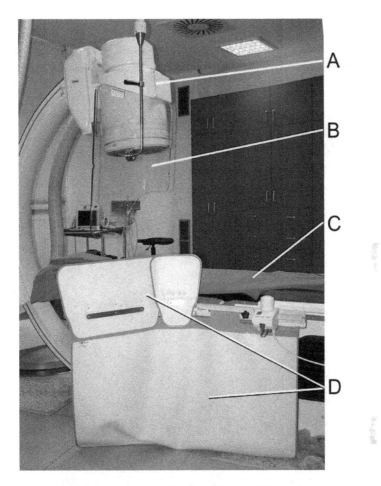

Figure 6. Radiation shields. Legend: A – image intensifier; B – Articulated, ceiling-mounted radiation protection screen; C – patient position; D – table-side shields.

The staff inside the cath lab must also wear the personal protection (fig. 7), which comes in several types and sizes. It is very important that one wears an adequate size protection garments. Firstly, lead apron should be worn. They come in different lead- or lead-equivalent thickness, and can weigh some 15 kg. It is advisable to wear the aprons which cover both the front and the back of the person. Because they may be heavy and put strain to the skeletal system, belts are used to take the weight off the shoulders. The minimum of protection is the equivalent of 0.5 mm of lead at the front. A two piece (blouse-plus-skirt design) is preferred by some operators. Another shield can be worn around the neck to protect the thyroid and neck tissues and organs (fig. 7). An additional small apron can be worn around the waist to increase the protection of the gonads (fig. 7). Since eyes can be affected when exposed to radiation over a prolonged period of time, it is advisable to wear leaded eyeglasses, or face-masks which are secured on the head (fig. 7). Protective eyewear must have at least the equivalent of protection of 0.5 mm of lead. Some recent investigations on the head exposure to radiation have resulted in a recommendation that leaded caps should also be worn.

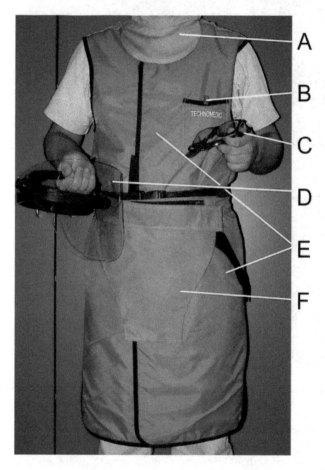

Figure 7. Personal protection for members of the staff in the cath lab. Legend: A –thyroid protection collar; B – outside personal dosimeter (in the pocket); C – protective eyeglasses; D – radiation panoramic full face mask for face shielding (preffered to eyeglasses); E – protective one-piece apron; F – additional protection for the gonads.

A cap with only 0.5 mm lead equivalence was proven to be more protective than a ceiling-mounted shield with 1.0 mm lead equivalence [21] This indicates that a significant amount of secondary scatter radiation, reflected from the walls of the cath lab, may reach the interventionist's head, despite the presence of a ceiling mounted lead glass shield, and this shield is actually designed to protect the operator's head from the primary scatter radiation from the patient. The annual head dose sustained by interventional cardiologists can be quite high, raising the issue of not only the cataract, but also brain tumors. The head dose may reach 60 mSv a year, and may in some cases exceed the occupational limit of 150 mSv a year recommended for the lens of the eye [22]. This information is the cause of the current consideration of the risks of radiation induced cataracts and malignancy, particularly brain cancer [23,24]. Primary scatter to the operator's unprotected head is highest for left anterior oblique (LAO) tube angulations [21]. However, some argue that a careful use of the lead glass shield provides similar protection of the operator's brain [20,25].

The exposure of the operator in general is higher when LAO projections are used, as opposed to RAO projections. The RAO positions are better regarding the operator dose, because the x-ray entrance point into the patient is kept away from the operator [3]. The RAO 90°, for example, exposes the interventionist to some three times less less scattered radiation than the usually used LAO 90° projection [26].

Even the line of interventonist's vision is important in this regard. The monitors in the cath lab are usually placed so that the patient can also follow the procedure, meaning that the monitors are to the interventionist's left front field of vision. For the operator, even leaning the head to the left increases the radiation exposure, and also the whole body posture is affected by this – the interventionist then stands closer to the x-ray tube, and to the source of scattered radiation. Just looking towards the tube exposes the lower parts of the face to levels 4–10 times greater than does looking rightwards [21]. Knowing that the monitor position typically determines the operator's predominant line of vision in interventional cardiology, it is advisable to place the monitors to the operator's right front side. By placing the monitors into the interventionist's right front part of the field of vision (fig. 5), radiation exposure of the interventonist's head can be dramatically reduced. This way, regardless of tube angulation, the lowest scatter towards the operator's head will occur in a line of vision toward the foot of the table. This means that in order to protect the eye lenses and the brain, interventional cardiologists should try to work with monitors positioned to the right [21]. Since the operator's hands might sometimes be directly under an x-ray beam, there are even sets of sterile leaded gloves (for single use, of course) that can be worn, although the material is obviously thicker than that used for normal sterile gloves, and the tactile feeling in the hands and at the operator's fingertips is not very precise.

The cath lab should be in a room of adequate size. Large rooms of some 60 m² are preferred not only because they are comfortable to work in, but also because in such rooms it is easy to employ the 'distance' and the 'shielding' principles of radiation protection [10]. A certain amount of space is also required for the ceiling-mounted radiation shields. Since the amount of radiation is reduced by the square distance from the source, in large rooms it is easy to distance and therefore protect oneself from radiation much better than in small rooms with limited space to move or stand. By staying inside the cath lab at the same time, assisting personnel can be readily available to attend the patient when needed.

The equipment used in cardio-angiology is some of the most sophisticated and complex used in medicine today. It must be well-maintained and the users must be well trained in using it. As stated before, in all modern cardiology units, each fluoroscopic image is captured using a short pulse of x-ray beam. The pulse itself lasts for 3-10 ms. Longer pulses would appear blurry since structures observed in cardiology move. The pulse rate is identical to the image capture rate, and between pulses no radiation is being produced. At pulse rate of 30 images per second, the human eye perceives the series of fast changing images as a seemingly continuous motion. However, the amount of radiation at this pulse rate might be excessive. Reducing the pulse rate by half reduces (roughly by half) the amount of radiation to the exposed persons, and slightly affects the sequence quality, but usually not as much as to negatively affect the procedure. For large patients who require larger amounts of radiation to penetrate their bodies, reduction of pulse rate can mean the difference between no skin injury and the occurrence of radiation burns. Dose-rate control can also be achieved through modulating pulse width, tube current, beam energy, and filtration, but not all of these parameters can be controlled by the operator sometimes. The optimal control of these parameters means that the interventionist will choose the dose-rate mode which gives the smallest amount of radiation, while at the same time enabling adequate image quality.

A very important factor in determining the amount of radiation which will be used is the size of the patients. Smaller patients demand less radiation, and the image is brighter, crisper, and with better contrast. Bigger patients, however, demand larger amounts of radiation to obtain the same image quality. That amount is further increased with steeply angulated projections, so the operator must be aware of this while working with larger patients, and choose the projections wisely, to adequately display the region of interest while, at the same time, maintain the lowest radiation dose possible. When the lesions are difficult to treat, that prolongs the beam-on time and doses can be extremely high. Positioning the patient on cardio-angiographic table also plays a role in radiation exposure. To protect the patient against radiation burns, and oneself from scattered radiation, the operator is advised to keep the patient higher, farther away from the radiation source, and at the same time closer to the image receptor [5,6,7].

4.4. Radiation dose monitoring

Today, the modern cardio-angiographic devices are equipped with dose-monitoring systems which record the amount of radiation and calculate the exposure of the patient. There are also simpler methods, such as film-monitoring in which a film layer is positioned beneath the patient, roughly at the site of the beam entrance. The film is sensitive to radiation and becomes darker with higher doses. It is examined after the procedure (or during the procedure if necessary), and a simple device estimates the exposure based on the degree of the film darkening. This method is very good for estimating the skin exposure when the beam enters from posterior, but lacks preciseness if very angulated or lateral projections are used.

Automated devices for exposure measurement usually measure air kerma. The unit of measurement is Gy. It is the sum of initial kinetic energies of all charged particles liberated by the x-rays per mass of air. This measures the amount of radiation at a point in space and can assess the level of hazard at the specified location. Most modern devices used in interventional cardiology have a built-in monitor of total accumulation of air kerma at a reference point, and this point in interventional cardiology approximates the position of the skin where the beam enters the patient. It adds up the radiation from all projections, making it in this sense more convenient than the film monitor, but it approximates, so the true result might be different from the measured value. Some machines have the possibility to measure kerma-area product and dose-area product. The logic of these devices is based on the fact that the beam area increases with the distance from the source, and the air kerma decreases. Theoretically, the product of these values is the same at all positions along the beam. This is primarily a quality control measurement, and if one wants to calculate the dose to the patient, usually a medical physicist must be consulted, because such calculations can be quite complicated.

As for the staff, radiation monitors must be worn at all times during the procedure. This way the exposure of the staff can be measured. It is necessary for interventional cardiologists and other personnel employed in the cath lab to wear personal radiation exposure monitors (dosimeters) on a regular basis, although sometimes this is not the case. Sometimes dosimeters are not worn because of a lack of awareness of risks associated with radiation and/or lack of education in radiation protection [27]. In some institutions or countries, regulatory bodies demand that the monitors are placed outside the protective aprons, while others demand that they must be worn underneath the protection garments. In some hospitals (as is the case in the hospital in which the author works), two monitors must be worn per person: one on the outside, and the other one beneath the protective apron. The one outside records the exposure of the unprotected areas (fig. 7). If only that one is worn, it can be approximated that the dose underneath 0.5 mm of lead equivalent is 0.5% of the dose measured on the outside monitor. Wearing only under-the-apron monitor may give the operator a false sense of security and lead to potentially heavy exposure of the unprotected body parts. Also, the monitoring of the exposure at the hands and legs/feet should be considered, at least periodically. Beside wearing the monitors, the staff working inside the radiation environment must undergo periodical clinical examinations to evaluate the state of their skin, to detect vision impairment, to do blood tests, and to check for chromosomal abnormalities, and possibly other diagnostic measures, as defined by the responsible regulatory bodies. Sometimes, if the doses of radiation exposure found in an employee are larger than recommended, the employee will be ordered to be removed from the radiation environment, temporarily or permanently.

5. Pregnancy and x-ray radiation in the cath lab

There are two ways in which the pregnancy can affect radiologic procedures in a cath lab: either one of the staff is pregnant, or the patient is pregnant. Both situations warrant a careful approach and need to be mentioned.

If a member of the staff is pregnant, different regulatory bodies define different forms of radiologic protection for the woman and the fetus. In some countries, the recommendations are that the fetus must be protected, while not interfering with the future mother's ability to do her job. The employees, both men and women, must be introduced to radiation safety measures in connection with reproductive issues. Usually, there is also a recommendation that all female employees of childbearing potential carry a whole-body dosimeter on the outside of the protective apron, as well as a dosimeter worn under the apron, at the abdominal level. The readings on these dosimeters must not exceed 0.25 mGy per month, thus ensuring that the conceptus receives less than a half of a maximum allowed dose recommended by the professional agencies (which is 0.5 mGy). A pregnant employee must be provided with an option to wear an additional pelvic shield of 0.25 to 0.5 mm of lead equivalent material. The employee should also be provided with duties involving less radiation exposure, if at all possible. In some countries, as is the case in the author's country, the pregnant employee who works in a medical radiation environment has the right to start pregnancy-leave at the very beginning of the pregnancy, and continue with it up to one year postpartum. It is the author's firm belief that all pregnant employees must be given an option to take pregnancy-leave as soon as they learn they are pregnant, so no unnecessary radiation risks, small as they might be, are imposed on the fetus and the pregnant mother-to-be.

When there is a pregnant patient in the cath lab, it is usually a patient with an acute coronary syndrome (ACS). Although pregnant women rarely have ACS, this is possible and the staff must be prepared for such an event. With general population, percutaneous coronary intervention (PCI) is the preferred treatment modality for an acute myocardial infarction. On the other hand, PCI in pregnancy includes the exposure of fetus to ionizing radiation. High doses of radiation carry the risk of a spontaneous abortion, fetal organ deformities, fetal mental retardation and a higher incidence of childhood cancer. However, radiation doses received by fetus during a PCI on a pregnant woman are completely acceptable and PCI can and must be performed in a pregnant woman with an ACS. Before the introduction of the practice of ACS treatment by using PCI, ACS mortality in pregnancy was as high as 20% [28]. Today, by using PCI in the treatment of ACS, the mortality from ACS in pregnancy is reduced to only 5% [29]. During the invasive cardiologic procedures, the x-ray beam is directed to the patient's chest. Some of the radiation does penetrate even to the fetus, and a part of it is scattered radiation from the mother's body. Contemporary cardio-angiography machines, with excellent beam collimation and a precise beam direction, have very little primary beam dissipation. Since that kind of radiation is still theoretically possible, it is mandatory to protect the pregnant patient's abdomen with protective leaded aprons. The mean exposure of a fetus during a PCI procedure is 0.02 mSv, and in very difficult and time-consuming procedures can reach up to 0.1 mSv. These doses are acceptable, and are even relatively small when compared to computer tomography (CT) scan of the abdomen (8 mSv on average, to a maximum of 49 mSv), pelvic CT scan (25 mSv on average, to a maximum of 79 mSv), abdominal radiography (1.4 mSv on average, with a maximum of up to 4.2 mSv), or even a CT-scan of the thorax (0.06 mSv on average, to a maximum of 0.96 mSv). Doses over 50-100 mSv increase the incidence of fetal malformation. The radiation which is scattered from the directly irradiated body part reaches the fetus, but this is only a small fraction of the radiation dose reaching the pregnant patient's thorax [5]. Although it protects from a direct beam, the leaded apron at the patient's abdomen will not protect the fetus from the scattered radiation within the patient's (pregnant woman's) body. Taken into account the spectre of causes of an acute myocardial infarction during pregnancy, PCI will in most cases be the treatment of choice during pregnancy. Not only that it treats the thromboembolic processes, but their causes can be treated also, namely the coronary dissection, which is a disproportionally common cause of ACS in pregnancy, probably because of the alterations in the connective tissue structure (including that within the coronary artery walls) mediated by pregnancy hormones. Once again, PCI is considered to be relatively safe during pregnancy, both for the pregnant patient and for the fetus and it must be employed as the first line of treatment for ACS in pregnancy because it dramatically reduces ACS mortality for pregnant women.

6. Conclusion

In conclusion, although the discovery of the x-ray radiation is more than 100 years old, the x-ray technology is developing as fast as ever. As much as we need to learn about its usefulness and the different forms of its application, we must always be aware of its dangers, risks, and limitations, and use it with care and adequately protect ourselves and our patients.

Author details

Jasmin Čaluk

BH Heart Center, Department of interventional cardiology, Tuzla, Bosnia and Herzegovina

References

[1] Novelline R. Squire's Fundamentals of Radiology. Harvard University Press. 5th edition. 1997.

[2] Tsapaki V, Maniatis PN, Magginas A et al.: What are the clinical and technical factors that influence the kerma-area product in percutaneous coronary intervention? Br. J. Radiol 2008;81:949-945.

[3] Saunamaki KI. Radiation Protection in the Cardiac Catheterization Laboratory. Interv Cardiol 2010;2(5):667-672.

[4] Cusma JT. X-Ray Cinefluorographic Systems. In: King SB & Yeung AC (eds.) Interventional Cardiology. The McGraw-Hill Companies, Inc, 2007.p109-119.

[5] Hirshfeld JW, Balter S, Brinker et al.: ACCF/AHA/SCAI Clinical competence statement on physician knowledge to optimize patient safety and image quality in fluoroscopically guided invasive cardiovascular procedures. Circulation 2005;111:511–532.

[6] Kuon E, Dahm JB, Robinson DM, et al: Radiation-reducing planning of cardiac catherization. Z. Kardiol 2005; 94: 663–673.

[7] Bashore TM: Radiation safety in the catherization laboratory. Am. Heart J 2004;147:375–378.

[8] Vano E, Gonzales L, Fernandez JM, et al: Influence of patient thickness and operation modes on occupational and patient radiation doses in interventional cardiology. Radiat. Prot. Dosimetry 2006;118:325–330.

[9] Reay J, Chapple CL, Kotre CJ: Is patient size important in dose determination and optimization in cardiology? Phys. Med. Biol 2003;48:3843–3850.

[10] Wagner LK. Operational Radiation Management for Patients and Staff. In: King SB & Yeung AC (eds.) Interventional Cardiology. The McGraw-Hill Companies, Inc, 2007.p121-135.

[11] Miller SW, Castronovo FP. Radiation exposure and protection in cardiac catheterisation laboratories.Am J Cardiol 1985;55:171–6.

[12] Yoshinaga S, Mabuchi K, Sigurdson AJ, et al. Cancer risks among radiologists and radiologic technologists: review of epidemiologic studies. Radiology 2004;233(2): 313-21.

[13] Wagner LK. Overconfidence, overexposure, and overprotection. Radiology. 2004;233(2):307-8.

[14] Venneri L, Rossi F, Botto N et al.: Cancer risk from professional exposure in staff working in cardiac catheterization laboratory: insights from the National Research Council's Biological Effects of Ionizising Radiation VII Report. Am. Heart J 2009;157:118–124.

[15] International Commission on Radiological Protection. ICRP Publication 85. Avoidance of radiation injuries from medical interventional procedures. Annals ICRP 2000;30(2). Oxford: Pergamon, Elsevier Science Ltd.

[16] Mercuri M, Xie C, Levy M, et al: Predictors of increased radiation dose during percutaneous coronary intervention. Am. J. Cardiol 2009;104:1241–1244.

[17] Caluk J, Osmanovic E, Barakovic F, et al. Direct coronary stenting in reducing radiation and radiocontrast consumption. Radiol Oncol 2010; 44(3): 153-157.

[18] Larrazet F, Dibie A, Philippe F, et al: Factors influencing fluoroscopy time and dose–area product values during ad hoc one-vessel percutaneous coronary angioplasty. Br. J. Radiol 2003;76:473–477.

[19] Miller DL, Vano E, Bartal G et al.: Occupational radiation protection in interventional radiology: a Joint Guideline of the Cardiovascular and and Interventional Radiology Society of Europe and the Society of Interventional Radiology. J Vasc Interv Radiol 2010;21(5):607-15.

[20] Shortt CP, Al-Hashimi H, Malone L, Lee MJ: Staff radiation doses to the lower extremities in interventional radiology. Cardiovasc. Interv. Radiol 2007;30:1206–1209.

[21] Kuon E, Birkel J, Schmitt M, Dahm JB. Radiation exposure benefit of a lead cap in invasive cardiology. Heart 2003;89:1205–1210.

[22] Renaud L. A 5-year follow up of the radiation exposure to in-room personnel during cardiac catheterization. Health Phys 1992;62:10–15.

[23] Folkerts KH, Münz A, Jung S. Estimation of radiation exposure and radiation risk to staff of cardiac catheterization laboratories. Z Kardiol 1997;86:258–63.

[24] Finkelstein MM. Is brain cancer an occupational disease of cardiologists? Can J Cardiol 1998;14:1385–8.

[25] Maeder M, Brunner-La Rocca HP, Wolber T et al.: Impact of lead glass screen on scatter radiation to eyes and hands in interventional cardiologists. Catheter. Cardiovasc. Interv 2006;67:18–23.

[26] Kuon E, Dahm JB, Empen K, et al: Identification of less-irradiating tube angulations in invasive cardiology. J. Am. Coll. Cardiol 2004;44:1420–1428.

[27] Niklason LT, Marx MV, Chan HP. Interventional radiologists: occupational radiation doses and risks. Radiology 1993;187:729–33.

[28] Roth A, Elkayam U. Acute myocardial infarction associated with pregnancy. Ann Intern Med. 1996;125(9):751-62.

[29] James AH, Jamison MG, Biswas MS et al.: Acute myocardial infarction in pregnancy: a United States population-based study. Circulation 2006;113(12):1564-1571.

Chapter 5

Non-Invasive Study of Coronary Circulation by Means of a Transthoracic Dipyridamole Stress Echocardiography with Coronary Flow Reserve Evaluation

Maurizio Turiel, Luigi Gianturco,
Vincenzo Gianturco and Bruno Dino Bodini

Additional information is available at the end of the chapter

1. Introduction

Ultrasound techniques represent easy and useful diagnostic tools able to detect cardiac morphological and functional damage.

Transthoracic echocardiography is a reliable, cheap and non-invasive technique that allows an accurate evaluation of valvular abnormalities, pericardial diseases and ventricular wall motion defects, while Doppler analysis is useful to study left ventricular diastolic filling, valvularfuctioning and pulmonary pressures. Rexhepaj et al [1] found significant differences in early diastolic flow velocity (E), atrial flow velocity (A) and E/A ratio in rheumatoid arthritis (RA) patients compared to the control group, suggesting that a subclinical impairment of left and right ventricular function is present in RA patients, when left ventricular thickness, dimensions and myocardial performance indexes were still normal.

A new clinical application of ultrasound imaging is represented by the transthoracic dipyridamole stress echocardiography with coronary flow reserve (CFR) evaluation. CFR is assessed in the distal left anterior descending coronary artery (LAD) defined by the ratio between peak diastolic velocity during stress and at baseline(Fig. 1-2). It is a highly sensitive (>90%) diagnostic marker for coronary artery disease (CAD)[2, 3] and, when associated with the evaluation of the regional wall motion analysis, it becomes also highly specific [4]. In literature reports, a value of CFR < 2 has been shown to accurately predict the presence of coronary stenosis. In absence of epicardial coronary stenosis, an abnormal CFR may reflect an impaired coronary microcirculation in patients with reperfused myocardial infarct, arterial hypertension with or without left ventricular hypertrophy, diabetes mellitus, hypercholesterolemia, syndrome X, hypertrophic cardiomyopathy and other diseases [5].The assessment of CFR has also a prognostic value, so that a reduced CFR correlates with a negative prognosis [6]. Recently, new evidence underlined that not only the binary (normal-abnormal) response in CFR but the continuous spectrum of CFR value is a strong independent prognostic predictor in patients with known or suspected CAD [7].

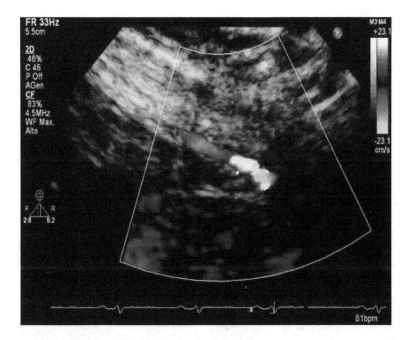

Figure 1. Distal left anterior descending (LAD) flow at color-Doppler.

Hirata et al [8] found a significant reduction of CFR in premenopausal women with SLE compared with age- and sex-matched controls. They concluded that microvascular impairment in SLE could be explained by functional alteration of endothelium which is responsible for the decrease vasodilation in response to pharmacological stress.

Turiel et al. 9 detected a significant impairment of CFR in 25 early RA patients, with disease duration less than 1 year and without any anti-rheumatic therapy. The reduced CFR in absence of wall motion abnormalities at rest and during pharmacological stress showed a coronary microcirculation involvement present in early RA and was associated with endothelial dysfunction.

Tissue Doppler Imaging (TDI) representsa new imaging modality which allows the measurement of myocardial velocities. Till now, TDI has been considered a reliable tool for the assessment of myocardial deformation, but this method is limited by angle-dependency and only deformation along the ultrasound beam can be derived from velocities, while myocardium deforms simultaneously in 3 dimensions [10]. Recently, Birdane et al [11] demonstrated that RA patients had a significant impairment of TDI biventricular diastolic functional parameters compared to healthy controls depending on age and use of steroids. To overcome TDI limitations, speckle tracking analysis has been introduced to evaluate myocardial strain along the longitudinal, circumferential and radial axis [12].

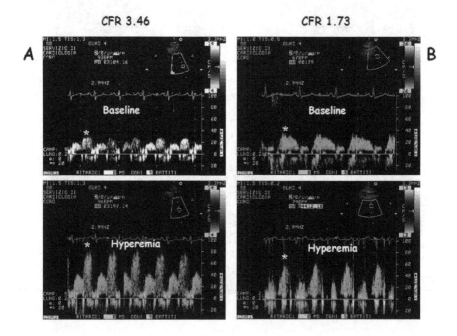

Figure 2. Doppler sampling of LAD: ratio between peak diastolic velocity during stress and at baseline.

Another very useful application of echocardiography in systemic autoimmune diseases is the echo transesophageal approach which is widely recognized as more sensitive than the transthoracic evaluation for the detection of valvular lesions [13] and identification of intracardiac masses.

In particular, Turiel et al [14] observed a large prevalence (61%) of valvular thickening or vegetations and/or potential embolic sources by transesophageal echocardiographic approach in 56 patients with primary antiphospholipid syndrome followed up for 5 years.

2. Utility of coronary flow reserve assessment in systemic autoimmune diseases

Patients suffering from systemic autoimmune diseases (SADs), especially RA, present higher risk of acute myocardial infarction and stroke [15], correlated with disease duration [16] with higher frequency of silent myocardial infarction and sudden death compared to general population [17]. This increase in cardiovascular (CV) risk seems not depending on traditional risk factors, thus suggesting a dominating role of RA-related risk factors [18, 19]. During these last years, attempts of explaining the accelerated atherosclerosis pathogenic pathways in RA were made; Attention particularly focused importance of chronic systemic inflammatory processwith high pro-inflammatory cytokines plasmatic levels. Presence of pro-atherogenic alterations such as dislipidemy, insulin-resistance, trombofilia and oxidative stress look favoring development of endothelial dysfunction that may be the initial stage of the atherosclerotic process [20, 21]. Arosio et al. [22], showed a reduced vasodilatation endothelium-dependant, changes in micro circle reactivity and an increased arterial stiffness in RA female patients.

Today non invasive evaluation of carotid median intimal thickness (IMT) is considered an early atherosclerosis clinical marker [23]. Kumeda et al. [24] observed in RA patients an increased IMT of common carotid and femoral artery, related to disease severity and duration. According to these evidences, Ciftci et al. [25] confirmed increased IMT and presence of reduced coronary flow reserve (CFR) in RA patients, correlating CV risk to disease duration. Moreover, Chung et al. [26], studied extension of coronary calcifications with CT, showing that patient with a long history of RA presents greater prevalence and severity of coronary calcifications compared to patients with early RA, also correlated with smoking and increase eritrosedimentation rate (ESR).

Nowadays, trans-thoracic echocardiographic evaluation of CFR by pharmacological stress (adenosine or dipyridamole)is considered a very useful exam as diagnose marker highly sensible (>90%) for coronary disease [27]. If associated with LV regional kinesis evaluation, acquires high specificity too. CFR value< 2 measured about at middle-distal tract of left anterior descending artery can accurately predict the presence of coronary significative stenosis. If epicardial vessels are free from significant stenosis a reduced CFR can be evidence of an alteration in coronary microcirculation in patients with reperfused myocardial infarction, high blood pressure with or without LV hypertrophy, diabetes mellitus, hypercholesterolemia, X syndrome, hypertrophic cardiomyopathy and collagen diseases. CFR measure has prognostic value in different pathologic conditions too[28].

Turiel et al. [29] showed a statistically significative variation of CFR among RA patients related with disease duration.

Endothelium function can be also studied through measure of asymmetric dymethilarginine(ADMA) plasmatic levels. Many clinical evidences support a close association between ADMA level and CV involvement in patients autoimmune diseases [30].

Higher ADMA plasmatic levels are reported in many conditions associated with high CV risk such as hypercholesterolemia, hypertriglyceridemia [31], peripheral artery disease [32], diabetes mellitus type II [33], acute coronary syndrome [34], chronic renal failure [35]. Moreover, Surdacki et al [36] evidenced in RA patient an association between high ADMA plasmatic levels and increased IMT at common carotid artery. Turiel et al. [37]observed an inverse correlation between ADMA and CFR in early stages of RA thus indicating a subclinical heart involvement already present at the beginning of the development of the disease.

Many clinical trials evidenced potential effects against atherosclerosis of therapies lead with disease modifying anti-rheumatic drugs (DMARDs), going beyond the simple control of inflammatory process and of disease activity (Tab. 1). In particular Hurlimann et al. [38] showed that anti-TNFα can not only reduce disease activity indexes, but also increase endothelial function in RA. Moreover, Sitia et al. [39] observed that long time treatment with DMARDs can reverse endothelial dysfunction, in early stages of disease.

Farmaco	Posologia	Tempo approssimativo per l' azione	Documentazione attività ref.	Costo per terapia annuale ($)
Idrossiclorochina	200 mg 2 volte al giorno	2 – 6 mesi	11,12	1.056
Oro intramuscolo	25-.50 mg i.m. ogni 2-4 sett	3 – 6 mesi	13	198
Azatioprina	50-150 mg al giorno	2 - 3 mesi	14	579 - 1.737
D-penicillamina	250-750 mg/die	3 – 6 mesi	15	865 - 2.595
Ciclosporina	25-4 mg/Kg/die	2 – 4 mesi	16	4.432 – 8.859
Methotrexate	7,5-20 mg/sett i.m o per os	1 – 2 mesi	17,18	orale 697 –1.859 i.m. 419 - 806
Sulfasalazina	100 mg 2-3 volte die	1 - 3 mesi	19 - 21	509 - 763
Leflunomide	20 mg al giorno	4 - 12 sett.	22,23	2.938
Infliximab (+ Methotrexate)	3-10 mg/Kg i.v. ogni 8 sett	da pochi giorni a 4 mesi	24 - 26	13.940 - 36.694
Etanercept	25 mg sc 2 volte/sett.	da pochi giorni a 4 sett.	27 - 29	15.436
Anakinra	100 mg sc quotidie	-	30,31	-

Table 1. Disease modifying anti-rheumatic drugs (DMARDs) in common use. (From American College of Rheumatology Subcommittee on Rheumatoid Arthritis Guidelines. Guidelines for the management of rheumatoid arthritis. Arthritis Rheum 2002; 46: 328-46, modified).

In addition, Mäki-Petäjä et al. [40] in a recent study confirmed the efficacy of associating ezetimibe and simvastatin in reducing the inflammatory process, but also in improving aortic stiffness in RA. Anyway, the possible validation of efficacy of the therapy with statin and/or biological drugs in modifying the evolution of atherosclerosis needs further perspective clinical trials.

3. Conclusions

Subclinical CV involvement related to specific and non-specific risk factors is frequent in systemic autoimmunity diseases. It begins rapidly after the onset of the disease and progresses with disease duration. All cardiac structures may be affected, and the cardiac complications include a variety of clinical manifestations. As CV involvement is associated with an unfavorable prognosis, the early detection of subclinical cardiac involvement in asymptomatic SADs patients is essential and then modern techniques nowhere existing and in this chapter illustrated are very very important to reach such goal.

Conflict of interest

None

Author details

Maurizio Turiel[1], Luigi Gianturco[1], Vincenzo Gianturco[2] and Bruno Dino Bodini[3]

*Address all correspondence to: maurizio.turiel@unimi.it

1 Cardiology Unit, IRCCS Galeazzi Orthopedic Institute, Department of Biomedical Sciences for Health, University of Milan, Milan, Italy

2 Department of Cardiovascular, Respiratory, Nephrological, Anesthesiological and Geriatrics Sciences, Sapienza University of Rome, Italy

3 Rehabilitation Unit, IRCCSGaleazzi Orthopedic Institute, Italy

References

[1] NoneRexhepaj N, Bajraktari G, Berisha I, Beqiri A, Shatri F, Hima F, Elezi S, Ndrepepa G. Left and right ventricular diastolic functions in patients with rheumatoid ar-

thritis without clinically evident cardiovascular disease. Int J Clin Pract 2006; 60: 683-688.

[2]   Caiati C, Zedda N, Montaldo C, Montisci R, Ruscazio M, Lai G, Cadeddu M, Meloni L, Iliceto S. Contrast-enhanced transthoracic second harmonic echo Doppler with adenosine: a noninvasive, rapid and effective method for coronary flow reserve assessment. J Am Coll Cardiol 1999; 34:122-130.

[3]   Hozumi T, Yoshida K, Ogata Y, Akasaka T, Asami Y, Takagi T, Morioka S. Non invasive assessment of significant left anterior descending coronary artery stenosis by coronary flow velocity reserve with transthoracic color Doppler echocardiography. Circulation 1998; 97: 1557-1562.

[4]   Rigo F, Richieri M, Pasanisi E, Cutaia V, Zanella C, Della Valentina P, Di Pede F, Raviele A, Picano E. Usefulness of coronary flow reserve over regional wall motion when added to dual-imaging dipyridamole echocardiography. Am J Cardiol 2003; 91: 269-273.

[5]   Dimitrow PP. Coronary flow reserve-measurement and application: focus on transthoracic Doppler echocardiography. Boston/Dordrecht/London: Kluwer Academic Publishers. 2002.

[6]   Rigo F, Gherardi S, Galderisi M, Pratali L, Cortigiani L, Sicari R, Picano E. The prognostic impact of coronary flow-reserve assessed by Doppler echocardiography in non-ischemic dilated cardiomyopathy. Eur Heart J 2006;27:1319-1323.

[7]   Cortigiani L, Rigo F, Gherardi S, Bovenzi F, Picano E, Sicari R. Implication of the continuous prognostic spectrum of Doppler echocardiographic derived coronary flow reserve on left anterior descending artery. Am J Cardiol 2010; 105:158-162.

[8]   Hirata K, Kadirvelu A, Kinjo M, Sciacca R, Sugioka K, Otsuka R, Choy A, Chow SK, Yoshiyama M, Yoshikawa J, Homma S, Lang CC. Altered coronary vasomotor function in young patients with Systemic Lupus Erythematosus. Arthritis and Rheum 2007; 56: 1904-1909.

[9]   Turiel M, Tomasoni L, Sitia S, Cicala S, Gianturco L, Ricci C, Atzeni F, De Gennaro Colonna V, Longhi M, Sarzi-Puttini P. Effects of long-term disease-modifying antirheumatic drugs on endothelial function in patients with early rheumatoid arthritis. Cardiovasc Ther. 2010 Oct;28(5):e53-64.

[10] Dandel M, Hetzer R. Echocardiographic strain and strain rate imaging – Clinical applications. Int J Cardiol 2009; 132: 11-24.

[11] Birdane A, Korkmaz C, Ata N, Cavusoglu Y, Kasifoglu T, Dogan SM, Gorenek B, Goktekin O, Unalir A, Timuralp B. Tissue Doppler imaging in the evaluation of the left and right ventricular diastolic functions in Rheumatoid Arthritis. Echocardiography 2007; 24: 485-493.

[12] Sitia S, Tomasoni L, Turiel M. Speckle tracking echocardiography: a new approach to myocardial function. World J Cardiol 2010; 2: 1-5.

[13] Turiel M, Muzzupappa S, Gottardi B, Crema C, Sarzi-Puttini P, Rossi E. Evaluation of cardiac abnormalities and embolic sources in primary antiphospholipid syndrome by transesophageal echocardiography. Lupus 2000;9: 406-412.

[14] Turiel M, Sarzi-Puttini P, Peretti R, Bonizzato S, Muzzupappa S, Atzeni F, Rossi E, Doria A. Five-year follow-up by transesophageal echocardiographic studies in primary antiphospholipid syndrome. Am J Cardiol 2005; 96: 574-579.

[15] Solomon DH, Goodson NJ, Katz JN, Weinblatt ME, Avorn J, Setoguchi S, Canning C, Schneeweiss S. Patterns of cardiovascular risk in rheumatoid arthritis. Ann Rheum Dis. 2006;65:1608-12.

[16] Solomon DH, Karlson EW, Rimm EB, Cannuscio CC, Mandl LA, Manson JE, Stampfer MJ, Curhan GC. Cardiovascular morbidity and mortality in women diagnosed with rheumatoid arthritis. Circulation. 2003;107:1303-7.

[17] Maradit-Kremers H, Crowson CS, Nicola PJ, Ballman KV, Roger VL, Jacobsen SJ, Gabriel SE. Increased unrecognized coronary heart disease and sudden deaths in rheumatoid arthritis: a population-based cohort study. Arthritis Rheum. 2005;52:402-11.

[18] Del Rincón ID, Williams K, Stern MP, Freeman GL, Escalante A. High incidence of cardiovascular events in a rheumatoid arthritis cohort not explained by traditional cardiac risk factors. Arthritis Rheum. 2001;44:2737-45.

[19] Del Rincón I, O'Leary DH, Freeman GL, Escalante A. Acceleration of atherosclerosis during the course of rheumatoid arthritis. Atherosclerosis. 2007;195:354-60.

[20] Voskuyl AE. The heart and the cardiovascular manifestations in rheumatoid arthritis. Rheumatology 2006;45:iv4-7.

[21] Dhawan SS, Quyyumi AA. Rheumatoid arthritis and cardiovascular disease. Curr Atheroscler Rep. 2008 Apr;10(2):128-33.

[22] Arosio E, De Marchi S, Rigoni A, Prior M, Delva P, Lech A. Forearm haemodynamics, arterial stiffness and microcirculatory reactivity in rheumatoid arthritis. J Hypertens. 2007;25:1273-8.

[23] Sidhu PS, Allen PL. Ultrasound assessment of internal carotid artery stenosis. Clin Radiol 1997;52: 654-8.

[24] Kumeda Y, Inaba M, Goto H, Nagata M, Henmi Y, Furumitsu Y, Ishimura E, Inui K, Yutani Y, Miki T, Shoji T, Nishizawa Y. Increased thickness of arterial intima-media detected by ultrasonography in patients with rheumatoid arthritis. Arthritis Rheum 2002; 46:1489-97.

[25] Ciftci O, Yilmaz S, Topcu S, Caliskan M, Gullu H, Erdogan D, Pamuk BO, Yildirir A, Muderrisoglu H. Imapired coronary microvascular function and increased intima-media thickness in rheumatoid arthritis. Atherosclerosis 2008; 198: 332-7.

[26] Chung CP, Oeser A, Raggi P, Gebretsadik T, Shintani AK, Sokka T, Pincus T, Avalos I, Stein CM. Increased coronary-artery atherosclerosis in rheumatoid arthritis. Arthritis Rheum 2005;52: 3045-53.

[27] Kerekes G, Soltész P, Nurmohamed MT, Gonzalez-Gay MA, Turiel M, Végh E, Shoenfeld Y, McInnes I, Szekanecz Z. Validated methods for assessment of subclinical atherosclerosis in rheumatology. Nat Rev Rheumatol 2012; 8(4): 224-34.

[28] Sitia S, Atzeni F, Sarzi-Puttini P, Di Bello V, Tomasoni L, Delfino L, Antonini-Canterin F, Di Salvo G, De Gennaro Colonna V, La Carrubba S, Carerj S, Turiel M. Cardiovascular involvement in systemic autoimmune diseases. Autoimmunity Rev 2009; 8: 281-286.

[29] Atzeni F, Sarzi-Puttini P, Delfino L, et al. Decreased coronary flow reserve in patients with rheumatoid arthritis. Ann Rheum Dis 2004;63:S196.

[30] De Gennaro Colonna V, Pascale V, Bianchi M, Ferrario P, Morelli F, Pascale W, Tomasoni L, Turiel M. Asymmetric dimethylarginine (ADMA): an endogenous inhibitor of nitric oxide sinthase and a novel cardiovascular risk molecole. Medical Science Monitor 2008; 15(4): 91-101.

[31] Lundman P, Eriksson MJ, Stuhlinger M, Cooke JP, Hamsten A, Tornvall P. Mild-to-moderate hypertriglyceridemia in young men is associated with endothelial dysfunction and increased plasma concentrations of asymmetric dimethylarginine. J Am Coll Cardiol 2001; 38: 111-6.

[32] Boger RH, Bode-Boger SM, Thiele W, Junker W, Alexander K, Frölich JC. Biochemical evidence for impaired nitric oxide synthesis in patients with peripheral arterial occlusive disease. Circulation 1997; 95:2068-74.

[33] Stuhlinger MC, Abbasi F, Chu JW, Lamendola C, McLaughlin TL, Cooke JP, Reaven GM, Tsao PS. Relationship between insulin resistance and an endogenous nitric oxide synthase inhibitor. JAMA 2002; 287: 1420-6.

[34] Bae SW, Stuhlinger MC, Yoo HS, Yu KH, Park HK, Choi BY, Lee YS, Pachinger O, Choi YH, Lee SH, Park JE. Plasma asymmetric dimethylarginine concentrations in newly diagnosed patients with acute myocardial infarction or unstable angina pectoris during two weeks of medical treatment. Am J Cardiol 2005;95: 729-33.

[35] MacAllister RJ, Rambausek MH, Vallance P, Williams D, Hoffmann KH, Ritz E. Concentration of dimethyl-l-arginine in the plasma of patients with end-stage renal failure. Nephrol Dial Transplant 1996; 11: 2449-52.

[36] Surdacki A, Martens-Lobenhoffer J, Wloch A, Marewicz E, Rakowski T, Wieczorek-Surdacka E, Dubiel JS, Pryjma J, Bode-Böger SM. Elevated plasma asymmetric dimethyl- L-arginine levels are linked to endothelial progenitor cell depletion and carotid atherosclerosis in rheumatoid arthritis. Arthritis Rheum 2007; 56: 809-19.

[37] Turiel M, Tomasoni L, Delfino L, Bodini B, Bacchiani G, Atzeni F, Sarzi-Puttini P, De Gennaro Colonna V. Clinical implications of assessing coronary flow reserve and

plasma asymmetric dimethylarginine in early rheumatoid arthritis. Eur J Echocardiogr 2007; 8: S35.

[38] Hurlimann D, Forster A, Noll G, Enseleit F, Chenevard R, Distler O, Béchir M, Spieker LE, Neidhart M, Michel BA, Gay RE, Lüscher TF, Gay S, Ruschitzka F. Anti-tumor necrosis factor-alpha treatment improves endothelial function in patients with rheumatoid arthritis. Circulation 2002; 106: 2184-7.

[39] Sitia S, Tomasoni L, Cicala S, Delfino L, Atzeni F, Sarzi-Puttini P, De Gennaro Colonna V, Turiel M. Effects of long-term disease-modifying antirheumatic drugs on endothelial function in patients with early rheumatoid arthritis. Eur J Echocardiogr 2008; 9:166.

[40] Mäki-Petäjä KM, Booth AD, Hall FC, Wallace SM, Brown J, McEniery CM, Wilkinson IB. Ezetimibe and simvastatin reduce inflammation, disease activity, and aortic stiffness and improve endothelial function in rheumatoid arthritis. J Am Coll Cardiol 2007; 50: 852-8.

Chapter 6

Computed Tomography Imaging of the Coronary Arteries

G.J. Pelgrim, M. Oudkerk and R. Vliegenthart

Additional information is available at the end of the chapter

1. Introduction

In this chapter the possibilities of computed tomography (CT) for imaging of the coronary arteries are examined. Only in the last decades CT has entered the field of cardiac imaging, due to technical developments. First the history of CT in cardiac imaging is described. When did this technique enter clinical practice and what level of temporal and spatial resolution does it reach nowadays?

The goal of the CT technique described in this chapter is to image the coronary arteries. It is important to know how a CT scan for coronary imaging is made. This is discussed in the second part of the chapter. Contraindications to coronary CT angiography (CCTA) are put forward followed by the explanation of scan acquisition techniques. A detailed overview is provided regarding different CCTA scan protocols and types of acquisitions.

One of the main disadvantages of CCTA is the patient exposure to radiation to acquire the imaging data. Therefore, an important goal in CCTA imaging is to reduce the radiation dose while maintaining diagnostic image quality. There are multiple developments in the area of CT radiation reduction, which are discussed in the next section.

The diagnostic accuracy of CCTA has been investigated extensively in recent years. In this section the diagnostic accuracy of different CT scanner generations for calcium scoring and CCTA are expanded upon. This includes results for different parameters used in diagnostic accuracy studies, such as sensitivity and specificity.

What are the indications for CCTA examinations? This is the question which is answered in the fifth section. While this is a dynamic field, the main indications, supported by different consensus statements, are discussed. Approximately ten indications are described and ordered by relevance. Examples of different indications are shown by patient CCTA images.

The future of cardiac CT is the last topic discussed. There are ample opportunities for future cardiac CT research such as CT perfusion imaging. These options are briefly mentioned.

2. Computed tomography

Computed tomography (CT) has been utilized in numerous fields in clinical practice since its invention in the 1970s. The first CT scanner was developed in 1971 by Geoffrey Hounsfield and installed at the Atkinson-Morley hospital in England. CT uses X-ray radiation to acquire 2D cross-sectional images of the body. X-ray imaging uses the different properties of different tissues to distinguish them in the image data. These images are acquired by a rapid 360 degree circular motion of the X-ray tube. The images are registered by the circular ray of X-ray detectors located in the gantry surrounding the patient. Then, a 2 dimensional reconstruction is made using the principle that an internal structure of the body can be made using multiple X-ray projections. To reconstruct a CT image, data from approximately 180^0 of gantry rotation are required. From the start in 1972, CT has had an important role in diagnostics as non-invasive imaging technique.

In cardiac imaging, however, CT did not gain ground until developments in recent years. Early CT modalities were limited in their ability to display cardiac morphological information due to the interference of cardiac motion and spatial resolution. The diameter of coronary arteries varies from large, 3 mm, to small, 1.5 mm. Therefore, the spatial resolution of the angiography technique should be at least 1 mm. [1] Temporal resolution was not sufficient to display the heart due to cardiac motion. Therefore, until recently, invasive coronary angiography (ICA) was the only accurate method for coronary imaging. [2, 3]

CT for cardiac imaging first entered the field with the development of electron beam computed tomography (EBCT) in the 1980s. EBCT was specifically developed for cardiac imaging, combining very high temporal resolution (50-100ms) with prospective electrocardiographic (ECG) triggering. The high temporal resolution combined with ECG triggering greatly reduced cardiac motion artifacts. The main clinical application of EBCT was the quantification of coronary calcium deposits in a so-called calcium score. The calcium score is correlated with degree and severity of coronary artery disease (CAD) and is a strong predictor of coronary events. [4, 5]The application of calcium scoring is explained in more detail further in this chapter. Main limitation of EBCT is the spatial resolution of between 1.5 mm and 3 mm in the z-axis. This prevents EBCT to accurately determine the severity of CAD, especially in CCTA setting. After the introduction of multidetector CT (MDCT) scanners in 1990s (see below) and due to limited availability of EBCT scanners, EBCT was used less frequently and eventually replaced by MDCT systems from 2003 onwards.

The developments in CT were rapid, compared to other imaging fields in the last decades. These developments have led to considerably improved temporal and spatial resolution. MDCT scanners use multiple detectors to acquire the data, scanning multiple detector rows in one rotation. Already 4- and 16-row MDCT scanners caused a revolution in cardiac imaging, however diagnostic accuracy in terms of specificity was generally low. [6-10] Sensitivity and negative predictive value were already good. MDCT proved useful in evaluation of coronary anomalies and bypass graft patency. Although the 16-row MDCT scanners had improved spatial resolution, making detection and characterization of coronary plaques and coronary wall changes possible, high heart rates, stents and severely calcified arteries, however, affected the image quality negatively. [11, 12]

In 2004, the next generation of MDCT scanners was introduced, with 32, 40 and 64 slices, another step forward in speed of volume coverage. Compared to 16-row MDCT scanners, the gantry rotation time of 64-row MDCT scanners improved from 500 ms to 330 ms. This translates in an improvement in temporal resolution from 250 ms to 165 ms, as only half a rotation is needed to acquire the data required for the image reconstruction. The visualization of the coronary arteries was again markedly improved, with a high sensitivity and specificity achieved for evaluation of coronary stenosis. [13-15] Examinations in patients with high heart rates were reported to still yield diagnostic images, with the use of multisegment reconstruction algorithms, reducing influence of motion artifacts. [16, 17]

Dual source computed tomography (DSCT) is one of the latest improvements in CT imaging modalities. The DSCT scanners consist of 2 tube-detector systems mounted in the same gantry, off-set by 90 degrees (perpendicular). Compared with conventional single-source CT scanners, the temporal resolution of this CT scanner is twice as high. This is because the temporal resolution is equal to a quarter of the gantry rotation. The other parameters, such as gantry rotation time, are equal to single-source CT scanners. In DSCT, the temporal resolution is further improved to 83 ms, further reducing the influence of motion artifacts on the image quality. Studies have shown an improvement in the assessment of the moving heart at a high heart rate without the need to use medication to control the heart rate during the examination. [18-22] Multiple studies have assessed the difference in image quality and accuracy of DSCT compared to 64-row scanners. [23-25] The higher temporal resolution resulted in better image quality and diagnostic accuracy.

Recent expansion of the detector width in MDCT has resulted in CT scanners with 256 and 320 detector rows. These systems allow for coverage of up to 320 slices during one rotation and in one heartbeat. This allows coverage of the whole heart in one gantry rotation. The principle of these CT scanners is the use of a cone beam. The X-ray tube can reach the detectors at the edges of the gantry readout, possibly displaying the whole heart in one scan. However, the 320-slice coverage comes at a cost as the temporal resolution is lowered to 350 ms and the edge of the scan range is prone to artifacts. [26-28]

The introduction of CT and different generations of CT scanners over time is described in Table 1. Continuously, new technologies are developed to improve the diagnostic performance of the CT technique for imaging the coronary arteries, including the spatial and temporal resolution.

Computed tomography development

Year	Technique
1971	First computed tomography scanner
1980s	Electron beam computed tomography (EBCT)
1990s	Multidetector CT scanner
2004	32-, 40-, 60-row multidetector CT
2006	Dual source computed tomography (DSCT)
2007	256- and 320-slice CT

Table 1. Development in computed tomography with highlights through the years

3. Imaging the coronary arteries by CCTA

The goal of coronary CT angiography (CCTA) is to image the coronary arteries, detect coronary artery calcification, and evaluate coronary stenosis or occlusion. Final aim is to aid the cardiologist in determining the best patient treatment and management.

High quality images are the most important prerequisite in the diagnostic assessment of the coronary arteries. Certain factors need to be taken into account to ensure a high-quality CCTA examination in the correct patient. These factors include selecting the right patients for the examination, proper patient preparation, an adequate CT scanner, optimal CT scan protocol, including synchronization of the CT data with the ECG information and proper reconstruction of image data, and dedicated software for evaluation of the coronary CT images. Furthermore, a prerequisite for CCTA is the injection of iodinated contrast material to delineate the lumen of the coronary arteries. Therefore, an absolute contraindication for CCTA is an allergy for iodine. An overview of contraindications for CCTA are listed in table 2. [29] Apart from general contraindications for CT, there are some specific contraindications for CCTA, such as high or irregular heart rates.

CCTA Contraindications

Atrial fibrillation (permanent or at time of the study)
Heart rate "/> 65 beats/minute refractory to heart-rate lowering agents
Bigeminy, Trigeminy, high degree heart block
Severe asthma
Creatinine "/> 1.8 (estimated Glomerular Filtration < 60), measurement of kidney function
Failed steroid preparation for contrast allergy
Morbid obesity (body mass index "/> 40)
Calcium score "/> 1000
Pregnancy
Inability to cooperate with scan acquisition and/or breath hold instructions

Table 2. Contraindications for coronary CTA

As stated before, motion artifacts on CCTA are observed more frequently in patients with higher and irregular heart rates. This negatively affects the image quality and reliability of detecting or excluding coronary stenoses. For earlier generation 16- to 64-row MDCT scanners it has been proven that the highest image quality is achieved in patients with a low heart rate (< 65 beats per minute). [30-32] It was shown that breath hold at end-inspiration reduces the heart rate by (on average) 6 beats per minute, which can be tested prior to performing the CCTA acquisition. In case of a patient's heart rate higher than 70 per minute it is advised to reduce the heart rate by medication. This can be done by administration of intravenous injection of 5-25 mg metoprolol.

Patients are positioned on the CT table in supine position. The three ECG leads are attached to the patient body to acquire an adequate ECG tracing, which is synchronized with the raw image data. Furthermore, an 18-gauge intravenous-line is inserted to ensure a correct injection of the contrast agent. The actual acquisition protocol consists of three steps: a topogram, a determination of the contrast arrival time using a test contrast bolus or acquisition of repetitive images during contrast injection for bolus tracking and the actual CCTA scan.

First, a low-energy topogram is acquired to enable accurate positioning of the scan volume. Afterwards, a non-contrast scan can be performed to obtain a coronary artery calcification (CAC) score. The coronary calcium score is a calculation of the amount of coronary artery calcium. The most commonly used method for coronary calcium quantification is the calcium score according to Agatston. [33] A negative CT scan for coronary calcium shows no calcification in the coronaries. A positive test means CAD is present, also when a patient is asymptomatic. The amount of calcification, expressed in the calcium score, can help to predict the risk of coronary events. The extent of CAD is graded according to the calcium, shown in table 3. The height of the calcium score is also strongly related to the risk of coronary heart disease. [34-37] At this moment, the strongest indication for coronary calcium scoring is in asymptomatic individuals at intermediate risk based on risk factors, to improve risk stratification. [38] For 64-row MDCT and earlier CT generations, a calcium score above 1000 is generally considered a contraindication for performing CCTA. The reason is twofold: patients with a very high calcium score have a considerable probability of having one or more significant stenosis, and severe calcifications cause blooming artifacts that limit the assessment of luminal narrowing.

Two techniques are available to correctly start the CCTA acquisition, based on arrival of contrast in the coronary arteries: the bolus tracking and the bolus timing technique. Bolus tracking involves a series of axial low-dose images to track the bolus of contrast material (every 2 seconds), monitoring the contrast enhancement in a region of interest (ROI) in the ascending aorta. The CCTA imaging sequence is initiated when the Hounsfield Unit (HU) in the ROI reaches a certain predefined level, usually 100 HU. The bolus timing technique involves an extra low-dose scan acquisition of a single slice. Here, a small contrast bolus followed by a saline flush is injected to determine the contrast arrival time. An axial low-dose image is generated every 2 seconds at a predefined ROI in the ascending aorta. The time between the start of the contrast injection and the arrival of contrast bolus in ROI is used as the scan delay for the actual CCTA. Both methods have similar results and have proven its usefulness in multiple research studies.

Cardiac calcium score	Extent of CAD, risk of coronary events in the next 5 year
0	No evidence of CAD, very low risk of coronary events
1-10	Minimal evidence of CAD, low risk of coronary events
11-100	Mild evidence of CAD, low-moderate risk of coronary events
101-400	Moderate evidence of CAD, moderate risk of coronary events
"/>400	Severe evidence of CAD, high risk of coronary events

Table 3. Cardiac calcium score related to the extent of CAD

When the correct volume and scan delay have been selected, the actual CCTA scan can be performed. A volume dataset of the coronary arteries is required, covering the entire heart. The scan is acquired during breath hold. A contrast agent with a high concentration of iodine is used (300mg/ml) to ensure adequate opacification of the coronary arteries. A total amount of 60-80 ml of contrast agent is injected with an injection speed of approximately 4-6 ml/s, which is flushed by a saline bolus of 40-70 ml (4-6 ml/s).

The scanning parameters are different from vendor to vendor and per scanner generation. These parameters are beyond the scope of this chapter and can be obtained from the vendor of the CT scanner.

CCTA scans are usually acquired in spiral mode, with continuous acquisition of data throughout the whole cardiac cycle (see Figure 1). The quality of the reconstructed axial images is determined by multiple parameters.

The use of retrospective ECG-triggering enables the reconstruction of CCTA images at different time points in the R-R interval. The R-R interval is the time between two R-tops in a normal cardiac cycle. In previous studies it has been shown that the optimal visualization window for coronary imaging, nearly free of motion artifacts is mid-diastole, at 60% to 70% of the R-R interval. In patients with higher or irregular heart rates however, better image quality is usually obtained at 25% to 35% of the R-R interval.

Slice thickness is dependent on the parameters of the specific CT scanner. Thinner slices improve the quality of the 3-dimensional dataset and the quality of the reconstructed images; on the downside it also increases the image noise which could potentially limit the diagnostic accuracy of the CCTA examination.

The CCTA images are usually reconstructed with a medium smooth reconstruction kernel. The reconstruction kernel, also referred to as 'filter' or 'algorithm' by some CT vendors, is one of the most important parameters affecting the image quality. In general, there is a tradeoff between the spatial resolution and noise for each kernel. Smooth kernels generate images with low noise, resulting in lower spatial resolution. A sharp kernel however, generates images with high spatial resolution but also have increased noise levels. [39] Recently, iterative reconstruction techniques have been introduced. These techniques reduce image noise by iteratively comparing the acquired image to a modeled projection. This algorithm is developed to reduce the radiation dose and enhance tube current modulation. These recon-struction techniques have shown to reduce image noise and improve image quality. [40, 41]

Prospective ECG-triggering is a technique used in cardiac CT that uses forward-looking pre-diction of R wave timing (see Figure 1). This is step-and-shoot non-spiral acquisition with-out table motion during imaging. Main advantage of prospective ECG-triggering is the lower radiation dose compared to retrospective ECG-triggering, see below. A disadvantage is the possibility of non-diagnostic coronary artery segments in case of unexpected changes or irregularity in the heart rate, as retrospective manipulation of the CT image data is gener-ally not possible. [42-44]

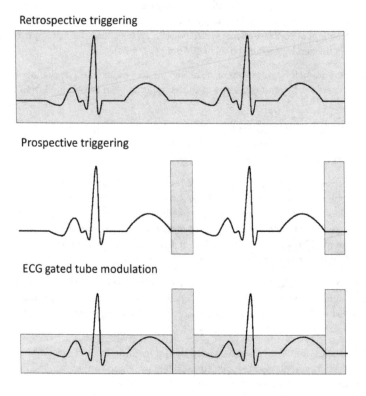

Figure 1. Different triggering techniques used to lower radiation dose. In retrospective triggering, the acquisition is constant and afterwards, the best cardiac phase is reconstructed for analysis. In prospective triggering, the acquisition is only performed during small parts of the cardiac phase, reducing radiation dose. In ECG-gated tube current modula-tion, the tube current is lowered during phases more likely to have motion artifacts and normal in the area of interest.

4. CCTA radiation exposure

The retrospectively ECG-gated CT is associated with relatively high radiation dose because of low pitch and overlapping data. Effective doses that have been published vary between 2 and 30 mSv, a prospective triggering mode has an effective radiation dose of between 1-3 mSv in adults. [42-45]

Radiation is a potential threat, which can cause harm to the human body. Therefore, minimizing radiation exposure to patients is of critical importance for physicians. The International Commission on Radiological Protection (ICRP) estimated that chance of acquiring fatal radiogenic cancer in the adult population is approximately 0.005%/mSv. Furthermore, it is assumed that there is no safe amount of radiation; any radiation amount is potentially harmful. Thus, effort should be taken to keep radiation doses as low as possible while maintaining diagnostic scan relevance. This radiological principle is also expressed as 'As Low As Reasonably Achievable' or ALARA. Multiple factors influence the radiation exposure, including scanner type, tube current, tube voltage, ECG triggering, high pitch helical scanning, scan range, slice thickness, acquisition time, overlap and pitch. Those factors influencing the radiation exposure should all be taken into account, minimizing the radiation to the lowest level possible.

Tube current can be modified according to the patient body mass index (BMI). Higher tube current increases the amount of photons per exposure time, reducing the image noise, but at the same time increasing the radiation dose. Patients with higher BMI need higher tube current to reduce the noise level, generated by the higher amount of tissue penetrated. The tube current should only be increased to a level necessary for acquiring adequate diagnostic images.

Increasing tube voltage will lead to higher energy X-ray beams with higher tissue penetration, and substantially increased radiation dose. Generally, 100 to 120 KeV tube voltages are sufficient for cardiac imaging. Only in really large patients, 140 KeV could be used. Reducing tube voltage will reduce radiation dose in proportion to the square of changes in tube voltage. [46, 47]

ECG synchronization is of particular importance for the amount of radiation exposure. As aforementioned, in retrospective ECG triggering data are acquired throughout the whole cardiac cycle and only the data with the least motion are used for reconstruction. In prospective ECG triggering, the tube is only activated during a predefined cardiac phase with presumably the greatest likelihood of minimal cardiac motion. Because there is no radiation exposure during the remainder of the cardiac cycle, this results in a dose reduction potential of 31%-86%. [25] In case of retrospective ECG triggering, ECG-based tube current modulation is an effective form of dose reduction (see Figure 1). This modulation utilizes the concept that coronary motion is least during end-systole and end-diastole. Therefore, the tube current is reduced by up to 96% during periods with presumably more cardiac motion and ramped up during diastole, when motion is at its lowest (for heart rates up to 65 bpm). [46] The image quality of phases with lower tube current is reduced, which is a downside of this technique. The potential dose reduction of ECG-gated tube current modulation is 13%-46%. [25].

The introduction of the second generation DSCT scanners made high-pitch helical scanning possible. This prospectively ECG triggered technique involves a high speed of the patient table. Due to this high pitch, the heart can be scanned in a fraction of one heartbeat. This eliminates overlapping volume coverage of sequential sections. Early results show dose reductions of up to 80% and CCTA examinations with <1 mSv radiation dose. [25]

Scan range is a term that indicates the z range (length) of the body which is scanned. Therefore, the larger the scan range is set, the higher the radiation exposure will be. The scan range should be limited to the range that is ultimately necessary to clarify the diagnostic questionnaire. A scan of the coronaries should not include the aortic root unless this is specifically asked by the referring physician. This will limit unnecessary radiation exposure.

Some factors of minor importance are slice thickness, acquisition time, overlap and pitch. Thinner slices will increase radiation dose because of the larger overlap and lower pitch, which increases acquisition time. The thinner slices need equal amounts of data to have same contrast-to-noise ratio compared to thicker slices. Because of this effect, the table speed needs to be slower with more overlap. This results in higher radiation exposure. With wider detector ranges and dynamic scanning, these factors become less important. A summary of important dose reduction parameters in CCTA is given in table 4.

The options to reduce radiation dose are numerous and radiation dose is gradually declining. As stated before, radiation dose of CTA acquisition over time ranges from 2 to 30 mSv. [45] In more recent scanners with optimal, up-to-date scanning protocols, the radiation dose will generally be around 3 to 4 mSv with a maximum of up to 7 mSv. [24, 25]

Radiation dose reduction
Scanner type (Multidetector, DSCT, etc.)
Tube current
Tube voltage
Triggering (Retrospective, prospective or ECG-gated tube current modulation)
High pitch helical scanning
Image reconstruction
Scan range
Slice thickness
Pitch
Overlap
Acquisition time

Table 4. Factors in radiation dose reduction

5. Diagnostic and prognostic accuracy

Scientific consensus documents have been published that address the appropriate use, diagnostic performance, prognostic value and interpretation of CCTA. [29, 48] Coronary artery calcium (CAC) is one of the parameters that can be assessed as part of a coronary CT acquisition protocol. As indicated, this involves a separate, non-contrast-enhanced CT scan prior to CCTA. The diagnostic and prognostic value of CAC was assessed in a systematic review by Sarwar et al. in 2009. [49] Only 146 of 25.903 asymptomatic individuals without CAC (0.56%) experienced a cardiovascular event during mean follow-up of 51 months. In 7 studies assessing the prognostic value of CAC in a symptomatic population, 1.8% of the patients without CAC had a cardiovascular event during mean follow-up of 42 months. Furthermore, the combined 18 studies indicated that the presence of CAC had a sensitivity and negative predictive value of 98% and 93%, respectively, for the detection of significant CAD on invasive coronary angiography. Prospective, population-based studies have shown that the calcium score is a very strong predictor of coronary events in asymptomatic individuals, with relative risks up to 10.

A systematic review and meta-analysis by Den Dekker et al. assessed the sensitivity and specificity of CCTA with 16-MDCT and newer CT scanner generations for significant stenosis at different degrees of coronary calcification. [50] 51 studies reported on the impact of calcium scoring on diagnostic performance of CCTA and were included the review. 27 out of 51 were suitable for the meta-analysis. Calcium scores were categorized as 0-100, 101-400, 401-1000, and >1000. On a patient-basis, sensitivity of CCTA for significant stenosis was 95.8%, 95.6%, 97.6% and 99.0%, respectively. Specificity of CCTA was 91.2%, 88.2%, 50.6% and 84.0%, respectively, for 64-row MDCT and newer scanners. The 16-row MDCT generation performed significantly worse than the more recently introduced scanners. Specificity was lower in the group with a calcium score of 401-1000, mainly because of low numbers of patients. These results suggest that even in severely calcified coronary arteries, the sensitivity and specificity of CCTA for significant stenosis is high, in case of 64-row MDCT or newer scanners. A cut-off for calcium scoring for CCTA in newer CT systems no longer seems necessary.

A systematic review and meta-analysis from 2007 by Abdulla et al. evaluated the diagnostic accuracy of 64-multidetector CT compared with conventional invasive coronary angiography (ICA) for coronary stenosis. [51] Mean sensitivity and specificity of CCTA to detect and exclude significant stenosis on a patient basis were 98% and 91% respectively. Single center studies have shown that the negative predictive value (NPV) of CCTA for 64-row MDCT scanners is high (>95%) and are clinically useful to rule out significant CAD. [15, 52, 53]

The diagnostic accuracy of ECG-gated 64-row MDCT in individuals without known CAD was assessed in a prospective multicenter trial named ACCURACY. [54] A total of 230 subjects underwent both CCTA and ICA. On a patient-based level the sensitivity, specificity, PPV and NPV to detect >50% stenosis were 95%, 83%, 64% and 99% respectively. The test characteristics for >70% stenosis were 94%, 83%, 48% and 99%, respectively. 64-row MDCT was shown to have a high diagnostic accuracy in detecting coronary stenosis, both at >50% and >70%. Even more importantly, the 99% NPV establishes CCTA as an alternative for ICA to rule out significant CAD.

Miller et al. (2008) also examined the accuracy of 64-row multidetector CT compared to conventional ICA. [55] In 291 patients with calcium score below 600, coronary segments with a diameter of >1.5 mm were analyzed by CCTA and ICA. 56% of the patients had obstructive CAD. Patient-based diagnostic accuracy of CCTA for ruling out stenosis >50% according to ICA revealed an area under the curve (AUC) of 0.93, with sensitivity, specificity, PPV, NPV of 85%, 90%, 91% and 83% respectively. The PPV and NPV in this study indicated that CCTA cannot replace ICA at that time.

Baumuller et al. compared CCTA with DSCT and 64-row MDCT in the diagnosis of significant coronary stenosis in 200 patients. [24] Of these patients, 100 underwent DSCT and 100 underwent MDCT. On a segment basis, sensitivity and specificity for DSCT were 96.4% and 97.4% respectively. For 64-row MDCT the sensitivity and specificity were 92.4% and 95.3% respectively. The NPV for DSCT and 64-row MDCT was 99.5% and 98.8% respectively. DSCT showed significantly improved accuracy and specificity for the diagnosis of significant stenosis on a segment basis, but shows comparable diagnostic accuracy compared to 64-row MDCT on a per patient-analysis.

In a study by Leber et al., DSCT was performed in 88 patients. [20] Results showed an overall sensitivity and specificity on a segment base of 95% and 90% respectively. DSCT accurately ruled out coronary stenosis in patients with intermediate pretest likelihood for CAD, independent of the heart rate. Higher heart rates did not show significant decrease in diagnostic accuracy.

A non-comprehensive overview of studies regarding the diagnostic accuracy of CT (64-row and DSCT) for significant stenosis versus ICA is shown in table 5. It can be concluded from most studies that CCTA has a good sensitivity, specificity and excellent NPV. Thus, CCTA can be used to rule out or detect the presence of CAD in selected symptomatic populations suspected of CAD.

Another important aspect of CCTA is the possibility to predict coronary events in symptomatic patients. This may have consequences for clinical management. Hulten et al. performed a systematic review and meta-analysis on the prognostic value of CCTA. In 18 studies 9.592 patients were evaluated with a median follow-up time of 20 months. [63] Major adverse cardiac events (MACE) occurred at an absolute rate of 0.6% (myocardial infarction (MI) or death) in patients with negative scan results. Occurrence of MACE in the positive scan group was 8.2%, with MI or death in 3.7%. Adverse cardiovascular events among patients with a normal CCTA are very rare and comparable to the baseline risks among healthy patients. The negative likelihood ratio of CCTA with normal findings is comparable to reported values for stress myocardial perfusion scans and stress echocardiography.

Author	Sensitivity (%)	Specificity (%)	PPV (%)	NPV (%)	Number of patients
Meijboom et al.[56]	99	64	86	97	360
Miller et al.[55]	85	90	91	83	291
Budoff et al.[54]	95	83	64	99	230
Baumuller et al.[24]	96.4	97.4	83.2	99.5	200
Tsiflikas et al.[57]	94	79	88	90	170
Sun et al.[58]	84.3	98.6	92.2	96.9	103
Ropers et al.[59]	98	81	79	99	100
Brodoefel et al.[19]	100	81.5	93.6	100	100
Weustink et al.[60]	99	87	96	95	100
Leber et al.[20]	95	90	74	99	88
Oncel et al.[53]	100	100	100	99	80
Raff et al.[15]	95	90	93	98	70
Ehara et al.[61]	98	86	98	86	69
Mollet et al.[52]	99	95	76	99	51
Achenbach et al.[62]	100	82	72	100	50
Johnson et al.[22]	100	89	89	100	35

Table 5. Accuracy of DSCT and 64-row CT in the detection of coronary stenosis on a segment level in comparison to ICA.

6. Indications

Even though CCTA has only become a viable potential alternative for ICA for selected patients since the development of 64-MDCT, already a number of indications are supported by scientific societies, and the number of indications is rapidly increasing. In 2008, a report of a writing group deployed by the Working Group Nuclear Cardiology and Cardiac CT of the European Society of Cardiology (ESC) and the European Council of Nuclear Cardiology (ECNC) was written with the indications, applications, limitations and training requirements for CCTA analysis. [64] In 2010, the American College of Cardiology Foundation (ACCF) along with key- and subspecialty societies conducted an appropriate use review of common clinical scenarios where CCTA is frequently considered and applied. [48] For potential clinical applications, the advantages and disadvantages of CCTA must be weighed against ICA. The following section lists the potential clinical indications for the use of CTA. This list starts with the strongest indication and reports to less frequent and less strong indications, taking different opinions of aforementioned societies into account.

The strongest indication for CCTA is to rule out significant luminal stenosis in stable patients with suspected CAD, at low-intermediate pretest likelihood of disease. As stated above, literature convincingly demonstrates that CCTA has a high negative predictive value and allows to reliably rule out CAD. [48, 64-66] Here, the aim is to avoid ICA when CT shows the absence of clinically relevant CAD. Based on clinical and statistical considerations, CCTA will be most useful in patients with an intermediate likelihood of CAD. The false-positive rate may be too high, for patients with a very low pretest likelihood. In patients with high pretest likelihood, it is not likely that a negative CT result excludes significant CAD.

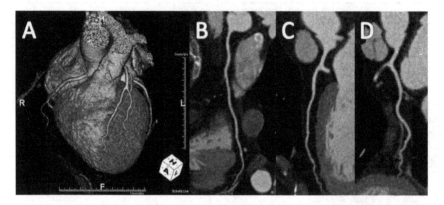

Figure 2. CCTA of a 61 year old women. A) 3D volume rendered reconstruction of the heart and the coronaries. The coronary arteries can be seen in the 3D reconstruction. B) Reconstruction of the right coronary artery (RCA) without CAD. C) Reconstruction of the left anterior descending artery of the same patient, also without stenosis. D) Circumflex (CX) reconstruction, not showing any disease.

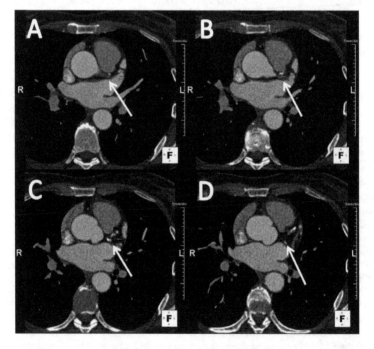

Figure 3. Overview of transverse CCTA images of a patient with an occlusion of the left main artery. In figs. A to C the arrow indicates the origin of the total occlusion. In image D the CX artery (retrograde filled) is pointed out.

Another application of CCTA is to rule out CAD in acute chest pain. This concerns patients presenting to the emergency room with acute chest pain, without direct evidence of myocardial infarction based on e.g. electrocardiogram or myocardial enzymes. In these patients, further testing is often necessary in order to rule out significant CAD, or prolonged observation in the emergency room. Coronary CTA has been found useful in these patients to rapidly assess the coronary arteries for the presence of luminal stenosis. Recent studies have shown the efficiency of applying CCTA in the emergency room. [67, 68]

CCTA can determine the complex course of anomalous coronary arteries. CCTA is the technique of choice for patient workup in known anomalous coronary vessels or vessels suspected to be anomalous because of the ease of data acquisition and the high resolution of the data set. CT has been qualified as an appropriate technique for evaluation of coronary anomalies. [48, 69-71] An example of CCTA analysis of coronary anomalies is shown in figure 4.

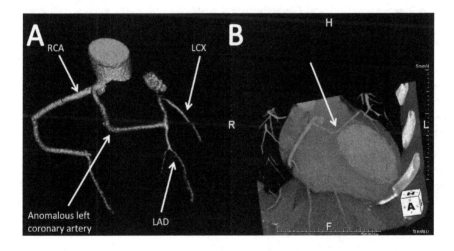

Figure 4. Patient with a coronary anomaly. A) The anomalous left coronary artery arises from the proximal RCA, through the septum into the LAD. B) Maximum intensity projection of the anomalous left coronary artery.

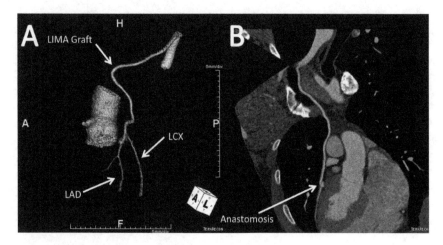

Figure 5. Evaluation after bypass-surgery, same patient as in figure 4. A) The distal left internal mammary artery (LI-MA) is anastomosed with the proximal LAD at the location of the former anomalous left coronary artery. B) The graft and distal LAD show good contrast filling.

Significant coronary artery disease, mainly left main disease, needs to be ruled out before non-coronary cardiac surgery. Cardiothoracic surgeons often request coronary angiography to rule out CAD in patients scheduled for cardiac surgery, for instance valve replacement. For this purpose, stress testing is not reliable enough, as ischemia could possibly be masked by the underlying pathology. CCTA may be a useful technique to analyze the coronary arteries, without having to perform an ICA. Meijboom et al. addressed the use of CCTA in the detection of CAD prior to aortic valve replacement. [72] The overall sensitivity and specificity of CCTA for detecting CAD was, respectively 100% and 82%. So, it can be assumed that patients scheduled for cardiac surgery can be evaluated by CCTA for the detection of CAD, without subgroups such as arrhythmias and unstable patients.

It has been determined that CCTA has a high accuracy for the detection of bypass graft stenosis and occlusion. [73-77] Bypass grafts are arteries or veins from elsewhere in the patient's body, grafted to the coronary arteries to bypass coronary stenosis and improve blood supply to the myocardium, shown in figure 5. Especially venous grafts have a larger diameter and are less prone to motion, which is an advantage for image quality. Coronary artery calcifications and dimensions of native coronary arteries complicate assessment of native coronary arteries in patients with bypass grafts. Recent studies showed that the sensitivity and specificity is lower in bypass graft patients. [75] Therefore, in clinical cases in which only bypass graft evaluation is required, CCTA use may be beneficial. If the coronary arteries also require assessment, value of CCTA will be limited.

Recent statements agree on the value of coronary calcium scoring in asymptomatic individuals at intermediate risk of cardiovascular disease. In these patients, the calcium score has shown to improve risk stratification compared to cardiovascular risk factors. [36, 37]

Multiple less frequent and less strongly supported applications for CCTA imaging are known. For instance, CTA can be used as an alternative when cardiac catheterization is impossible or carries too much risk. Percutaneous coronary intervention (PCI) planning could also be an indication for CCTA. CT can more reliably identify parameters influencing PCI outcome such as length and extent of the stenosis than ICA. [78] Assessment of coronary stent lumen is also a possibility with CCTA. The ability to assess the stents depends on many factors including stent type and diameter.

CCTA Indications
Detection of CAD in symptomatic patients with suspected CAD
Detection of CAD in asymptomatic individuals without known CAD
Detection of CAD in a newly diagnosed heart failure without known CAD
Rule out CAD before non-coronary cardiac surgery
Clarify unclear findings in other noninvasive imaging techniques
Assessment post CABG (Graft evaluation)
Assessment post PCI (Stent evaluation)
Evaluation of anomalies of coronary arterial and thoracic arteriovenous vessels
Evaluation of complex adult congenital heart disease
Evaluation of ventricular morphology and systolic function

Table 6. Table Indications for CCTA analysis

7. Potential new application

It is important to realize that the presence of a significant stenosis on CCTA does not equate with hemodynamically significant CAD. Not all stenoses result in reduced myocardial perfusion in stress, and not all patients with a positive ischemia test have coronary stenosis. Thus, whereas angiographic evaluation of coronary artery pathology (morphological information) is needed on the one hand, assessment of inducible ischemia (functional information) due to coronary narrowing is necessary on the other hand. The number of different examinations that a patient has to undergo may be considerably reduced by combining morphological and functional data acquisition in one technique. CT, PET/CT and SPECT/CT have the potential of providing both functional and morphological information. [79] CT perfusion imaging is still early in development. It has different imaging options such as dynamic perfusion CT and (static) dual energy CT. Dynamic perfusion CT acquires multiple images of the contrast buildup in the myocardium, which can be monitored. Myocardial segments perfused by a stenotic artery will have a slower and lower contrast upslope resulting in a hypodense area in the myocardium. In dual-energy imaging, the amount of iodine contrast in the myocardium can be derived based on images at different KeV energy levels, an indication of blood distribution in the myocardium.

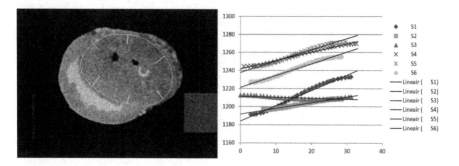

Figure 6. Dynamic CT perfusion analysis in a pig heart. The heart is divided into 6 segments (5 white lines and 1 blue line). Mean attenuation over time is monitored. B) Upslope of contrast enhancement in the 6 different segments in HU (not corrected for baseline -1024). Segments S2 and S3 have significantly lower upslope, corresponding with an applied stenosis in the CX artery.

8. Conclusion

Recent advances in modern CT technique have established CCTA as an accepted modality for coronary angiography in specific patients groups. One of the most important uses of CCTA is to exclude significant CAD in symptomatic patients at low-intermediate probability of significant stenosis. To yield most benefit from CCTA, patient selection remains important. Appropriate use will largely depend on patient characteristics, for instance pre-test likelihood of CAD. The advances in CT scanner technology have reduced the concerns about radiation dose, an important prior disadvantage. Exciting new imaging techniques in cardiac CTA could evolve in a comprehensive test for the assessment of CAD, making analysis of both anatomy and function possible in one modality.

Author details

G.J. Pelgrim[1,2*], M. Oudkerk[2] and R. Vliegenthart[1,2]

*Address all correspondence to: g.j.pelgrim@umcg.nl

1 Department of Radiology, University of Groningen, University Medical Center Groningen, Groningen, Netherlands

2 Center for Medical Imaging – North East Netherlands, University of Groningen, University Medical Center Groningen, Groningen, Netherlands

References

[1] Dodge JT, Jr., Brown BG, Bolson EL, Dodge HT. (1992) Lumen diameter of normal human coronary arteries. Influence of age, sex, anatomic variation, and left ventricular hypertrophy or dilation. Circulation; 86: 232-46.

[2] Harell GS, Guthaner DF, Breiman RS et al. (1977) Stop-action cardiac computed tomography. Radiology; 123: 515-7.

[3] Ritman EL, Kinsey JH, Robb RA et al. (1980) Three-dimensional imaging of heart, lungs, and circulation. Science; 210: 273-80.

[4] Keelan PC, Bielak LF, Ashai K et al. (2001) Long-term prognostic value of coronary calcification detected by electron-beam computed tomography in patients undergoing coronary angiography. Circulation; 104: 412-7.

[5] Guerci AD, Spadaro LA, Goodman KJ et al. (1998) Comparison of electron beam computed tomography scanning and conventional risk factor assessment for the prediction of angiographic coronary artery disease. Journal of the American College of Cardiology; 32: 673-9.

[6] Achenbach S, Giesler T, Ropers D et al. (2001) Detection of coronary artery stenoses by contrast-enhanced, retrospectively electrocardiographically-gated, multislice spiral computed tomography. Circulation; 103: 2535-8.

[7] Nieman K, Oudkerk M, Rensing BJ et al. (2001) Coronary angiography with multislice computed tomography. Lancet; 357: 599-603.

[8] Achenbach S. (2004) Detection of coronary stenoses by multidetector computed tomography: it's all about resolution. Journal of the American College of Cardiology; 43: 840-1.

[9] Flohr TG, Schoepf UJ, Kuettner A et al. (2003) Advances in cardiac imaging with 16-section CT systems. Academic radiology; 10: 386-401.

[10] Kuettner A, Trabold T, Schroeder S et al. (2004) Noninvasive detection of coronary lesions using 16-detector multislice spiral computed tomography technology: initial clinical results. Journal of the American College of Cardiology; 44: 1230-7.

[11] Stein PD, Beemath A, Kayali F et al. (2006) Multidetector computed tomography for the diagnosis of coronary artery disease: a systematic review. The American journal of medicine; 119: 203-16.

[12] Herzog C, Britten M, Balzer JO et al. (2004) Multidetector-row cardiac CT: diagnostic value of calcium scoring and CT coronary angiography in patients with symptomatic, but atypical, chest pain. European radiology; 14: 169-77.

[13] Pugliese F, Mollet NR, Runza G et al. (2006) Diagnostic accuracy of non-invasive 64-slice CT coronary angiography in patients with stable angina pectoris. European radiology; 16: 575-82.

[14] Ong TK, Chin SP, Liew CK et al. (2006) Accuracy of 64-row multidetector computed tomography in detecting coronary artery disease in 134 symptomatic patients: influence of calcification. American heart journal; 151: 1323 e1-6.

[15] Raff GL, Gallagher MJ, O'Neill WW, Goldstein JA. (2005) Diagnostic accuracy of noninvasive coronary angiography using 64-slice spiral computed tomography. Journal of the American College of Cardiology; 46: 552-7.

[16] Herzog C, Nguyen SA, Savino G et al. (2007) Does two-segment image reconstruction at 64-section CT coronary angiography improve image quality and diagnostic accuracy? Radiology; 244: 121-9.

[17] Wintersperger BJ, Nikolaou K, von Ziegler F et al. (2006) Image quality, motion artifacts, and reconstruction timing of 64-slice coronary computed tomography angiography with 0.33-second rotation speed. Investigative radiology; 41: 436-42.

[18] Flohr TG, McCollough CH, Bruder H et al. (2006) First performance evaluation of a dual-source CT (DSCT) system. European radiology; 16: 256-68.

[19] Brodoefel H, Burgstahler C, Tsiflikas I et al. (2008) Dual-source CT: effect of heart rate, heart rate variability, and calcification on image quality and diagnostic accuracy. Radiology; 247: 346-55.

[20] Leber AW, Johnson T, Becker A et al. (2007) Diagnostic accuracy of dual-source multi-slice CT-coronary angiography in patients with an intermediate pretest likelihood for coronary artery disease. European heart journal; 28: 2354-60.

[21] Klepzig H. (2008) Diagnostic accuracy of dual-source multi-slice CT-coronary angiography in patients with an intermediate pretest likelihood for coronary artery disease. European heart journal; 29: 680.

[22] Johnson TR, Nikolaou K, Busch S et al. (2007) Diagnostic accuracy of dual-source computed tomography in the diagnosis of coronary artery disease. Investigative radiology; 42: 684-91.

[23] Nakashima Y, Okada M, Washida Y et al. (2011) Evaluation of image quality on a per-patient, per-vessel, and per-segment basis by noninvasive coronary angiography with 64-section computed tomography: dual-source versus single-source computed tomography. Japanese journal of radiology; 29: 316-23.

[24] Baumuller S, Leschka S, Desbiolles L et al. (2009) Dual-source versus 64-section CT coronary angiography at lower heart rates: comparison of accuracy and radiation dose. Radiology; 253: 56-64.

[25] Fink C, Krissak R, Henzler T et al. (2011) Radiation dose at coronary CT angiography: second-generation dual-source CT versus single-source 64-MDCT and first-generation dual-source CT. AJR American journal of roentgenology; 196: W550-7.

[26] Mizuno N, Funabashi N, Imada M et al. (2007) Utility of 256-slice cone beam tomography for real four-dimensional volumetric analysis without electrocardiogram gated acquisition. International journal of cardiology; 120: 262-7.

[27] Dewey M, Zimmermann E, Deissenrieder F et al. (2009) Noninvasive coronary angiography by 320-row computed tomography with lower radiation exposure and maintained diagnostic accuracy: comparison of results with cardiac catheterization in a head-to-head pilot investigation. Circulation; 120: 867-75.

[28] Rybicki FJ, Otero HJ, Steigner ML et al. (2008) Initial evaluation of coronary images from 320-detector row computed tomography. The international journal of cardiovascular imaging; 24: 535-46.

[29] Abbara S, Arbab-Zadeh A, Callister TQ et al. (2009) SCCT guidelines for performance of coronary computed tomographic angiography: a report of the Society of Cardiovascular Computed Tomography Guidelines Committee. Journal of cardiovascular computed tomography; 3: 190-204.

[30] Pugliese F, Mollet NR, Hunink MG et al. (2008) Diagnostic performance of coronary CT angiography by using different generations of multisection scanners: single-center experience. Radiology; 246: 384-93.

[31] Hoffmann MH, Shi H, Manzke R et al. (2005) Noninvasive coronary angiography with 16-detector row CT: effect of heart rate. Radiology; 234: 86-97.

[32] Sun Z, Choo GH, Ng KH. (2012) Coronary CT angiography: current status and continuing challenges. The British journal of radiology; 85: 495-510.

[33] Agatston AS, Janowitz WR, Hildner FJ et al. (1990) Quantification of coronary artery calcium using ultrafast computed tomography. Journal of the American College of Cardiology; 15: 827-32.

[34] Budoff MJ, Shaw LJ, Liu ST et al. (2007) Long-term prognosis associated with coronary calcification: observations from a registry of 25,253 patients. Journal of the American College of Cardiology; 49: 1860-70.

[35] Greenland P, Bonow RO, Brundage BH et al. (2007) ACCF/AHA 2007 clinical expert consensus document on coronary artery calcium scoring by computed tomography in global cardiovascular risk assessment and in evaluation of patients with chest pain: a report of the American College of Cardiology Foundation Clinical Expert Consensus Task Force (ACCF/AHA Writing Committee to Update the 2000 Expert Consensus Document on Electron Beam Computed Tomography). Circulation; 115: 402-26.

[36] McClelland RL, Chung H, Detrano R et al. (2006) Distribution of coronary artery calcium by race, gender, and age: results from the Multi-Ethnic Study of Atherosclerosis (MESA). Circulation; 113: 30-7.

[37] Elias-Smale SE, Proenca RV, Koller MT et al. (2010) Coronary calcium score improves classification of coronary heart disease risk in the elderly: the Rotterdam study. Journal of the American College of Cardiology; 56: 1407-14.

[38] Piers LH, Salachova F, Slart RH et al. (2008) The role of coronary artery calcification score in clinical practice. BMC cardiovascular disorders; 8: 38.

[39] Achenbach S, Boehmer K, Pflederer T et al. (2010) Influence of slice thickness and reconstruction kernel on the computed tomographic attenuation of coronary atherosclerotic plaque. Journal of cardiovascular computed tomography; 4: 110-5.

[40] Leipsic J, Labounty TM, Heilbron B et al. (2010) Adaptive statistical iterative reconstruction: assessment of image noise and image quality in coronary CT angiography. AJR American journal of roentgenology; 195: 649-54.

[41] Scheffel H, Stolzmann P, Schlett CL et al. (2012) Coronary artery plaques: cardiac CT with model-based and adaptive-statistical iterative reconstruction technique. European journal of radiology; 81: e363-9.

[42] Gutstein A, Wolak A, Lee C et al. (2008) Predicting success of prospective and retrospective gating with dual-source coronary computed tomography angiography: development of selection criteria and initial experience. Journal of cardiovascular computed tomography; 2: 81-90.

[43] Huang B, Li J, Law MW et al. (2010) Radiation dose and cancer risk in retrospectively and prospectively ECG-gated coronary angiography using 64-slice multidetector CT. The British journal of radiology; 83: 152-8.

[44] Hirai N, Horiguchi J, Fujioka C et al. (2008) Prospective versus retrospective ECG-gated 64-detector coronary CT angiography: assessment of image quality, stenosis, and radiation dose. Radiology; 248: 424-30.

[45] Hausleiter J, Meyer T, Hermann F et al. (2009) Estimated radiation dose associated with cardiac CT angiography. JAMA : the journal of the American Medical Association; 301: 500-7.

[46] Hausleiter J, Meyer T, Hadamitzky M et al. (2006) Radiation dose estimates from cardiac multislice computed tomography in daily practice: impact of different scanning protocols on effective dose estimates. Circulation; 113: 1305-10.

[47] Siegel MJ, Schmidt B, Bradley D et al. (2004) Radiation dose and image quality in pediatric CT: effect of technical factors and phantom size and shape. Radiology; 233: 515-22.

[48] Taylor AJ, Cerqueira M, Hodgson JM et al. (2010) ACCF/SCCT/ACR/AHA/ASE/ASNC/NASCI/SCAI/SCMR 2010 appropriate use criteria for cardiac computed tomography. A report of the American College of Cardiology Foundation Appropriate Use Criteria Task Force, the Society of Cardiovascular Computed Tomography, the American College of Radiology, the American Heart Association, the American Soci-

ety of Echocardiography, the American Society of Nuclear Cardiology, the North American Society for Cardiovascular Imaging, the Society for Cardiovascular Angiography and Interventions, and the Society for Cardiovascular Magnetic Resonance. Journal of the American College of Cardiology; 56: 1864-94.

[49] Sarwar A, Shaw LJ, Shapiro MD et al. (2009) Diagnostic and prognostic value of absence of coronary artery calcification. JACC Cardiovascular imaging; 2: 675-88.

[50] den Dekker MA, de Smet K, de Bock GH et al. (2012) Diagnostic performance of coronary CT angiography for stenosis detection according to calcium score: systematic review and meta-analysis. European radiology.

[51] Abdulla J, Abildstrom SZ, Gotzsche O et al. (2007) 64-multislice detector computed tomography coronary angiography as potential alternative to conventional coronary angiography: a systematic review and meta-analysis. European heart journal; 28: 3042-50.

[52] Mollet NR, Cademartiri F, van Mieghem CA et al. (2005) High-resolution spiral computed tomography coronary angiography in patients referred for diagnostic conventional coronary angiography. Circulation; 112: 2318-23.

[53] Oncel D, Oncel G, Tastan A, Tamci B. (2007) Detection of significant coronary artery stenosis with 64-section MDCT angiography. European journal of radiology; 62: 394-405.

[54] Budoff MJ, Dowe D, Jollis JG et al. (2008) Diagnostic performance of 64-multidetector row coronary computed tomographic angiography for evaluation of coronary artery stenosis in individuals without known coronary artery disease: results from the prospective multicenter ACCURACY (Assessment by Coronary Computed Tomographic Angiography of Individuals Undergoing Invasive Coronary Angiography) trial. Journal of the American College of Cardiology; 52: 1724-32.

[55] Miller JM, Rochitte CE, Dewey M et al. (2008) Diagnostic performance of coronary angiography by 64-row CT. The New England journal of medicine; 359: 2324-36.

[56] Meijboom WB, Meijs MF, Schuijf JD et al. (2008) Diagnostic accuracy of 64-slice computed tomography coronary angiography: a prospective, multicenter, multivendor study. Journal of the American College of Cardiology; 52: 2135-44.

[57] Tsiflikas I, Brodoefel H, Reimann AJ et al. (2010) Coronary CT angiography with dual source computed tomography in 170 patients. European journal of radiology; 74: 161-5.

[58] Sun ML, Lu B, Wu RZ et al. (2011) Diagnostic accuracy of dual-source CT coronary angiography with prospective ECG-triggering on different heart rate patients. European radiology; 21: 1635-42.

[59] Ropers U, Ropers D, Pflederer T et al. (2007) Influence of heart rate on the diagnostic accuracy of dual-source computed tomography coronary angiography. Journal of the American College of Cardiology; 50: 2393-8.

[60] Weustink AC, Meijboom WB, Mollet NR et al. (2007) Reliable high-speed coronary computed tomography in symptomatic patients. Journal of the American College of Cardiology; 50: 786-94.

[61] Ehara M, Surmely JF, Kawai M et al. (2006) Diagnostic accuracy of 64-slice computed tomography for detecting angiographically significant coronary artery stenosis in an unselected consecutive patient population: comparison with conventional invasive angiography. Circulation journal : official journal of the Japanese Circulation Society; 70: 564-71.

[62] Achenbach S, Goroll T, Seltmann M et al. (2011) Detection of coronary artery stenoses by low-dose, prospectively ECG-triggered, high-pitch spiral coronary CT angiography. JACC Cardiovascular imaging; 4: 328-37.

[63] Hulten EA, Carbonaro S, Petrillo SP et al. (2011) Prognostic value of cardiac computed tomography angiography: a systematic review and meta-analysis. Journal of the American College of Cardiology; 57: 1237-47.

[64] Schroeder S, Achenbach S, Bengel F et al. (2008) Cardiac computed tomography: indications, applications, limitations, and training requirements: report of a Writing Group deployed by the Working Group Nuclear Cardiology and Cardiac CT of the European Society of Cardiology and the European Council of Nuclear Cardiology. European heart journal; 29: 531-56.

[65] Hamon M, Biondi-Zoccai GG, Malagutti P et al. (2006) Diagnostic performance of multislice spiral computed tomography of coronary arteries as compared with conventional invasive coronary angiography: a meta-analysis. Journal of the American College of Cardiology; 48: 1896-910.

[66] Vanhoenacker PK, Heijenbrok-Kal MH, Van Heste R et al. (2007) Diagnostic performance of multidetector CT angiography for assessment of coronary artery disease: meta-analysis. Radiology; 244: 419-28.

[67] Meijboom WB, van Mieghem CA, Mollet NR et al. (2007) 64-slice computed tomography coronary angiography in patients with high, intermediate, or low pretest probability of significant coronary artery disease. Journal of the American College of Cardiology; 50: 1469-75.

[68] Hoffmann U, Truong QA, Schoenfeld DA et al. (2012) Coronary CT angiography versus standard evaluation in acute chest pain. The New England journal of medicine; 367: 299-308.

[69] Hollander JE, Litt HI, Chase M et al. (2007) Computed tomography coronary angiography for rapid disposition of low-risk emergency department patients with chest pain syndromes. Academic emergency medicine : official journal of the Society for Academic Emergency Medicine; 14: 112-6.

[70] Deibler AR, Kuzo RS, Vohringer M et al. (2004) Imaging of congenital coronary anomalies with multislice computed tomography. Mayo Clinic proceedings Mayo Clinic; 79: 1017-23.

[71] Datta J, White CS, Gilkeson RC et al. (2005) Anomalous coronary arteries in adults: depiction at multi-detector row CT angiography. Radiology; 235: 812-8.

[72] Meijboom WB, Mollet NR, Van Mieghem CA et al. (2006) Pre-operative computed tomography coronary angiography to detect significant coronary artery disease in patients referred for cardiac valve surgery. Journal of the American College of Cardiology; 48: 1658-65.

[73] Nieman K, Pattynama PM, Rensing BJ et al. (2003) Evaluation of patients after coronary artery bypass surgery: CT angiographic assessment of grafts and coronary arteries. Radiology; 229: 749-56.

[74] Meyer TS, Martinoff S, Hadamitzky M et al. (2007) Improved noninvasive assessment of coronary artery bypass grafts with 64-slice computed tomographic angiography in an unselected patient population. Journal of the American College of Cardiology; 49: 946-50.

[75] Ropers D, Pohle FK, Kuettner A et al. (2006) Diagnostic accuracy of noninvasive coronary angiography in patients after bypass surgery using 64-slice spiral computed tomography with 330-ms gantry rotation. Circulation; 114: 2334-41; quiz

[76] Salm LP, Bax JJ, Jukema JW et al. (2005) Comprehensive assessment of patients after coronary artery bypass grafting by 16-detector-row computed tomography. American heart journal; 150: 775-81.

[77] Feuchtner GM, Schachner T, Bonatti J et al. (2007) Diagnostic performance of 64-slice computed tomography in evaluation of coronary artery bypass grafts. AJR American journal of roentgenology; 189: 574-80.

[78] Mollet NR, Hoye A, Lemos PA et al. (2005) Value of preprocedure multislice computed tomographic coronary angiography to predict the outcome of percutaneous recanalization of chronic total occlusions. The American journal of cardiology; 95: 240-3.

[79] Flohr TG, Klotz E, Allmendinger T et al. (2010) Pushing the envelope: new computed tomography techniques for cardiothoracic imaging. Journal of thoracic imaging; 25: 100-11.

Chapter 7

Clinical and Research Applications of Optical Coherence Tomography Imaging in Coronary Artery Disease

Takao Hasegawa and Kenei Shimada

Additional information is available at the end of the chapter

1. Introduction

Optical coherence tomography (OCT) is an optical analog of intravascular ultrasound (IVUS) that allows microscopic visualization of coronary plaque types and intracoronary tissue. The high-resolution images of OCT produce an intense interest in adopting this imaging technique for both clinical and research purposes.

In clinical aspects, OCT imaging for undergoing percutaneous coronary intervention (PCI) is feasible and provides superior resolution of arterial pathology than IVUS. During PCI, OCT can assess pre-procedural coronary plaque morphology and acute effects of coronary intervention (dissection, tissue prolapse, thrombi, and incomplete stent apposition (ISA)). Moreover, OCT provides more useful information to consider PCI strategy, such as distal protection, optimal stent landing zone.

In research aspects, OCT provides characterization of coronary plaque to assess factors associated with acute coronary syndrome (ACS) and vessel healing process after stent implantation. Recent studies have shown that OCT is useful for the assessment of coronary atherosclerotic plaques (plaque rupture, erosion, thin-cap fibroatheroma (TCFA), and intracoronary thrombi) in patients with ACS. In addition, OCT can detect the proliferation of vasa vasorum and the distribution of macrophages surrounding vulnerable plaques. OCT provides cardiologists with the tool they need to better understand the pathological condition of ACS.

According to vessel healing after stent implantation, OCT can provide stent strut coverage, ISA, and restenotic tissue characteristics at follow up. Previous OCT studies have shown that delayed neointimal coverage after drug-eluting stent (DES) implantation vs. bare metal stent (BMS) implantation. Pathological studies have indicated that the proportion of delayed neointimal coverage represents the best morphometric predictor of late stent thrombosis. Recent OCT studies demonstrate that restenotic tissue characteristics is completely different between BMS and DES. Therefore, OCT can play an important role to assess the safety profile of novel DES systems.

Finally, we introduce usefulness of 3-dimensional reconstruction of the OCT images and 1-μm resolution OCT.

2. Differences between IVUS and OCT

OCT is an optical analog of IVUS, used to examine the coronary arteries. There is a pressing need for improved characterization of coronary pathology to better recognize the factors associated with coronary vessel disease and to guide the selection of better interventional strategies. The resolution and contrast of OCT is attractive for these applications and suitable catheters to access the coronary arteries in detail. There are several differences between IVUS and OCT, as shown in Table 1 [1]. The resolution of OCT (10-20 μm) is 10-fold higher than that of IVUS (100-150 μm), but the penetration depth is lower with OCT (1-2 mm) than with IVUS (4-8 mm) [2]. According to other important difference between IVUS and OCT, the removal of blood is not need for IVUS examination but OCT examination. To examine coronary arteries, blood must first be removed during an OCT examination because of the strong attenuation of light by blood [3].

OCT imaging uses an interferometry technique based on time-delay measurements of the light reflected or backscattered from the tissues [4]. We can use two processing modes used for intracoronary OCT imaging, the first generation time-domain OCT (TD-OCT) imaging systems and the more recently available second generation frequency-domain OCT (FD-OCT) imaging systems [5, 6].

The first-generation OCT (ImageWire and M2/3 OCT system; LightLab Imaging, Inc., Westford, Massachusetts) incorporated both an OCT imaging wire and an over-the-wire occlusion balloon. To deliver the image wire and remove blood from the target lesion, an over-the-wire occlusion balloon catheter was used. The OCT imaging procedure started with advancing a 0.014-inch coronary guide wire distal to the target lesion. The occlusion catheter is passed along the guide wire through the lesion. After the guide wire and OCT image wire were exchanged, the occlusion balloon is pulled back proximal to the lesion. Then, ringer's solution was continuously flushed at 0.5–0.6 ml/s through the occlusion catheter lumen using a power injector, and the balloon was inflated to 0.3–0.5 atm by an inflation device to block blood flow. When an OCT image well appeared, a motorized pullback was initiated from the imaging system console. The first-generation OCT was not user-friendly and had several disadvantages of complex procedure, such as balloon occlusion and relatively short length of image acquisition due to the limited frame rate. To improve these disadvantage, a new generation of OCT systems, termed FD-OCT imaging methods, has been developed.

FD-OCT imaging methods, utilize a light source with variable wavelength that is tuned to continuously oscillate between 1250 and 1350 nm, a so-called wavelength swept laser, instead of the broadband light source used in TD-OCT. As a result, FD-OCT system can enable faster image acquisition and greater scan depths compared with TD-OCT system. Intravascular OCT examination has been frustrated by requiring blood removal. However, FD-OCT system can enable faster image acquisition and greater scan depths compared with TD-OCT system. As a result, only intermittent injection of transparent fluid through guiding catheter for a few seconds enables to obtain entire coronary images [6, 7]. FD-OCT system has been developed (Dragonfly imaging catheter and C7- XR OCT system; LightLab Imaging, Inc., St Jude Medical,St Paul, Minnesota, USA). Differences between TD- (M3) and FD-OCT (C7-XR) systems are shown in Table 1 [8]. This advance may provide dramatic improvements in understanding coronary atherosclerosis and response to intravascular interventions such as angioplasty and stenting.

3. Clinical applications of OCT imaging

In clinical aspects, OCT imaging for undergoing PCI is feasible and provides superior resolution of arterial pathology than intravascular ultrasound. During PCI, OCT can assess pre-procedural coronary plaque morphology.

Regarding to plaque characterization, OCT can differentiate three types of coronary plaques, such as fibrous, calcified, and lipid-rich. Fibrous plaque is characterized by a homogenous high signal region with low attenuation, calcified plaque by a well-delineated, low-signal region with sharp borders, and lipid-rich plaques as a low-signal region with diffuse borders [9]. Importantly, a histology-controlled OCT study showed >90% sensitivity and specificity for detecting lipid-rich plaque in comparisons with pathological specimens. [9, 10]. Moreover, OCT can recognize vulnerable plaques, such as plaque rupture, erosion, intracoronary thrombus, TCFA.

Assessment of plaque characteristics before PCI is useful to choose optimal interventional strategy. Tanaka et al. showed that TCFA was often observed at target lesions of the patients with no reflow after PCI compared with good reflow (50% versus 16%, $P = 0.005$). The frequency of the no reflow phenomenon increased according to the lipid arc assessed by OCT [11]. When OCT detects lipid-rich plaque and TCFA especially in patients with ACS, we should consider to use distal protection devices to prevent no-reflow phenomenon.

Another aspect, plaque type at the stent edges has an impact on the occurrence of edge dissections. Gonzalo et al. showed that presence of edge dissection was significantly more frequent when the plaque type at the edge was fibrocalcific (43.8%) or lipid rich (37.5%) than when the plaque was fibrous (10%) [12]. This study demonstrated that complex plaque type at the stent edge might influence on the presence of edge dissections from OCT observation. The OCT guide stenting might be a useful assistance to achieve optimal landing zone.

After PCI, OCT can assess acute effects of coronary intervention (dissection, tissue prolapse, and ISA). Dissection, tissue prolapse, and ISA were observed more often with OCT than with IVUS [13, 14]. Coronary dissection is frequently observed at the distal stent edge because of the oversized stent diameter or complex types of plaque at the stent edge by OCT. When there is no limited coronary flow by angiography and adequate area of the true lumen by OCT, no additional procedure might be necessary for the treatment of coronary dissection [15].

There are 2 types of tissue prolapse, plaque prolapse or thrombus prolapse. OCT can distinguish between plaque prolapse and thrombus prolapse. Plaque prolapse is characterized by smooth surface with no signal attenuation, and thrombus protrusion by irregular surface with significant signal attenuation. Minor tissue prolapse identified by IVUS was not found to be associated with angiographic in-stent restenosis [16]. However, the relationship tissue prolapse identified by OCT and angiographic in-stent restenosis has not been elucidated.

ISA by OCT was identified as clear separation between at least one stent strut and the vessel wall. To check the stent apposition to the vessel wall, the distance between surface of stent strut and adjacent inatima border should be measured because of differences of stent and polymer thickness [8]. Small ISA, which is detected by only OCT but not by IVUS, could disappear by neointimal growth during follow-up period [15].

4. Research applications of OCT imaging

In research aspects, OCT can provide characterization of coronary plaque to assess factors associated with ACS and vessel healing process after stent implantation.

The first OCT study to assess in vivo culprit lesion morphology in patients with ACS showed that higher frequency of TCFA in ACS compared with stable angina pectoris (72% in acute myocardial infarction (AMI), 50% in unstable angina pectoris, and 20% in stable angina pectoris; $P = 0.012$) [2]. Kubo et al. showed superiorities of TD-OCT for the detection of plaque rupture (73% vs. 40% vs. 43%, $P = 0.021$), erosion (23% vs. 0% vs. 3%, $P = 0.003$), and thrombus (100% vs. 33% vs. 100%, $P < 0.001$) compared with IVUS and coronary angioscopy in patients with AMI [17]. The frequency of vulnerable plaque (plaque rupture, erosion, and thrombus) by detected OCT was similar to that of the pathological reports. As described above, OCT is more useful to assess atherosclerotic plaque instability compared to other intracoronary imaging devices.

OCT has been proposed as a high resolution imaging modality that can identify vasa vasorum as microchannels with tiny black holes (50-100 μm). The proliferation of vasa vasorum has been identified recently as a common feature of vulnerable plaque [18]. Kitabata et al. demonstrated increase of microvessels counts in TCFA [19]. An observational study of OCT revealed that the presence of microvessels in the plaques was also associated with positive remodeling and elevated high-sensitive C-reactive protein levels [19]. The OCT evaluation of microvessels counts might be helpful for assessing plaque vulnerability.

Moreover, the other unique aspect of OCT is the detection of macrophages. Degradation of the fibrous cap matrix by macrophages is associated with atherosclerotic plaque instability

[20]. Macrophages detected by OCT were observed as a 'bright spot', with a high signal variance from the surrounding tissue. Tearney et al. [21] and MacNeill et al. [16] descried OCT is capable to evaluate cap macrophage content accurately. High degree of positive correlation was observed between OCT and histological measurements of macrophage density in fibrous cap ($r < 0.84$, $P < 0.0001$). OCT provided to detect a cap macrophage density $> 10\%$ with 100% sensitivity and specificity [19].

According to vessel healing after stent implantation, OCT can provide stent strut coverage, ISA, and restenotic tissue characteristics at follow up. Previous OCT studies have shown that delayed neointimal coverage after DES implantation vs. BMS implantation [22]. Pathological studies have indicated that the proportion of delayed neointimal coverage represents the best morphometric predictor of late stent thrombosis [23, 24]. Recent OCT studies demonstrate that restenotic tissue characteristics is completely different between BMS and DES [21, 25]. Therefore, OCT can play an important role to assess the safety profile of novel DES systems.

5. Future directions of OCT imaging

Recently, a second-generation OCT technology, termed FD-OCT, has been developed that solves the TD-OCT limitations by imaging at much higher frame rates with slightly deeper penetration depth and greater scan area. In combination with a short, non-occlusive flush and rapid spiral pullback, the higher frame rates generated by FD-OCT enable imaging of the 3-dimensional reconstruction of longer segments of coronary arteries. The 3-dimensional OCT can express all of the coronary microanatomy and pathology previously visualized by OCT, including lipid pools, calcium, macrophages, thin fibrous caps, cholesterol crystals, thrombus, stent, and stents with neointimal hyperplasia [26]. The 3-dimensional OCT may be useful as a research tool for assessing human coronary pathophysiology and as a clinical tool for guiding the management of coronary artery disease.

Progress in understanding, diagnosis, and treatment of coronary artery disease has been hindered because of inability to observe cells and extracellular components associated with human coronary atherosclerosis *in situ*. A µOCT system with a very broad bandwidth light source and common-path spectral-domain OCT technology provides 1-µm axial resolution ranging in tissue [27]. The µOCT is possible to visualize many key cellular and subcellular features relevant to atherogenesis, plaque rupture, thrombosis, and neointimal healing after stenting *in situ*. The µOCT technology has the potential to make a significant impact in cardiovascular pathology.

6. Conclusion

The high resolution of OCT provides histology-grade definition of the microstructures of coronary atherosclerosis in vivo. Introduction of this attractive imaging method contributes significant progression in both clinical and research aspects. Clinically, OCT can provide more useful information to consider PCI strategy for getting the optimal interventional results. On the other hand, OCT is a useful imaging device for understanding, diagnosis, and treatment of coronary artery disease. In the future direction of OCT systems, 3-dimensional OCT and µOCT may be upcoming in the field of coronary artery disease. These novel OCT technologies will play an important role for investigation of coronary artery disease.

	IVUS	TD-OCT (M3)	FD-OCT (C7)
Axial resolution, µm	100-150	15-20	12-15
Lateral resolution, µm	150-300	39	19
Frame rate, fps	30	20	100
Pullback speed, mm/s	0.5-2.0	0.5-2.0	10-25
Scan diameter, mm	8-10	6.8	10
Penetration depth, mm	4-8	1-2	1-2
Balloon occlusion	Unnecessary	Necessary	Unnecessary

IVUS, intravascular ultrasound; OCT, optical coherence tomography; TD, time-domain; FD, frequency-domain; fps, frames per second.

Modified from Terashima M et al, korean j intern med 2012;27:1-12.

Table 1. Differences among IVUS, TD-OCT, and FD-OCT

	IVUS	OCT
Dissection	○	◉
Tissue prolapse	△	◉
ISA	○	◉
Stent expansion	◉	○
Lesion coverage	○	○

IVUS, intravascular ultrasound; OCT, optical coherence tomography; ISA, incomplete stent apposition.

Table 2. Acute effects of coronary intervention between IVUS and OCT

Author details

Takao Hasegawa and Kenei Shimada

*Address all correspondence to: shimadak@med.osaka-cu.ac.jp

Department of Internal Medicine and Cardiology, Osaka City University Graduate School of Medicine, Abeno-ku, Osaka, Japan

References

[1] Yamaguchi T, Terashima M, Akasaka T, Hayashi T, Mizuno K, Muramatsu T, et al. Safety and feasibility of an intravascular optical coherence tomography image wire system in the clinical setting. The American journal of cardiology. 2008;101(5):562-7.

[2] Jang IK, Tearney GJ, MacNeill B, Takano M, Moselewski F, Iftima N, et al. In vivo characterization of coronary atherosclerotic plaque by use of optical coherence tomography. Circulation. 2005;111(12):1551-5. Epub 2005/03/23.

[3] Kataiwa H, Tanaka A, Kitabata H, Imanishi T, Akasaka T. Safety and usefulness of non-occlusion image acquisition technique for optical coherence tomography. Circulation journal : official journal of the Japanese Circulation Society. 2008;72(9):1536-7.

[4] Huang D, Swanson EA, Lin CP, Schuman JS, Stinson WG, Chang W, et al. Optical coherence tomography. Science. 1991;254(5035):1178-81.

[5] Suter MJ, Nadkarni SK, Weisz G, Tanaka A, Jaffer FA, Bouma BE, et al. Intravascular optical imaging technology for investigating the coronary artery. JACC Cardiovascular imaging. 2011;4(9):1022-39.

[6] Yun SH, Tearney GJ, Vakoc BJ, Shishkov M, Oh WY, Desjardins AE, et al. Comprehensive volumetric optical microscopy in vivo. Nature medicine. 2006;12(12):1429-33.

[7] Imola F, Mallus MT, Ramazzotti V, Manzoli A, Pappalardo A, Di Giorgio A, et al. Safety and feasibility of frequency domain optical coherence tomography to guide decision making in percutaneous coronary intervention. EuroIntervention : journal of EuroPCR in collaboration with the Working Group on Interventional Cardiology of the European Society of Cardiology. 2010;6(5):575-81.

[8] Terashima M, Kaneda H, Suzuki T. The role of optical coherence tomography in coronary intervention. The Korean journal of internal medicine. 2012;27(1):1-12.

[9] Yabushita H, Bouma BE, Houser SL, Aretz HT, Jang IK, Schlendorf KH, et al. Characterization of human atherosclerosis by optical coherence tomography. Circulation. 2002;106(13):1640-5.

[10] Kume T, Akasaka T, Kawamoto T, Watanabe N, Toyota E, Neishi Y, et al. Assessment of coronary arterial plaque by optical coherence tomography. The American journal of cardiology. 2006;97(8):1172-5.

[11] Tanaka A, Imanishi T, Kitabata H, Kubo T, Takarada S, Tanimoto T, et al. Lipid-rich plaque and myocardial perfusion after successful stenting in patients with non-ST-segment elevation acute coronary syndrome: an optical coherence tomography study. European heart journal. 2009;30(11):1348-55.

[12] Gonzalo N SP, Okamura T, Shen ZJ, Garcia-Garcia HM, Onuma Y, van Geuns RJ, Ligthart J, Regar E. Relation between plaque type and dissections at the edges after

stent implantation: an optical coherence tomography study. Int J Cardiol 2011;150(2): 151-5.

[13] Bouma BE, Tearney GJ, Yabushita H, Shishkov M, Kauffman CR, DeJoseph Gauthier D, et al. Evaluation of intracoronary stenting by intravascular optical coherence tomography. Heart. 2003;89(3):317-20.

[14] Diaz-Sandoval LJ, Bouma BE, Tearney GJ, Jang IK. Optical coherence tomography as a tool for percutaneous coronary interventions. Catheterization and cardiovascular interventions : official journal of the Society for Cardiac Angiography & Interventions. 2005;65(4):492-6.

[15] Kume T, Okura H, Miyamoto Y, Yamada R, Saito K, Tamada T, et al. Natural history of stent edge dissection, tissue protrusion and incomplete stent apposition detectable only on optical coherence tomography after stent implantation - preliminary observation. Circulation journal : official journal of the Japanese Circulation Society. 2012;76(3):698-703.

[16] Hoffmann R, Mintz GS, Dussaillant GR, Popma JJ, Pichard AD, Satler LF, et al. Patterns and mechanisms of in-stent restenosis. A serial intravascular ultrasound study. Circulation. 1996;94(6):1247-54.

[17] Kubo T, Imanishi T, Takarada S, Kuroi A, Ueno S, Yamano T, et al. Assessment of culprit lesion morphology in acute myocardial infarction: ability of optical coherence tomography compared with intravascular ultrasound and coronary angioscopy. Journal of the American College of Cardiology. 2007;50(10):933-9.

[18] Kolodgie FD, Gold HK, Burke AP, Fowler DR, Kruth HS, Weber DK, et al. Intraplaque hemorrhage and progression of coronary atheroma. The New England journal of medicine. 2003;349(24):2316-25.

[19] Kitabata H, Tanaka A, Kubo T, Takarada S, Kashiwagi M, Tsujioka H, et al. Relation of microchannel structure identified by optical coherence tomography to plaque vulnerability in patients with coronary artery disease. The American journal of cardiology. 2010;105(12):1673-8. Epub 2010/06/12.

[20] Moreno PR, Falk E, Palacios IF, Newell JB, Fuster V, Fallon JT. Macrophage infiltration in acute coronary syndromes. Implications for plaque rupture. Circulation. 1994;90(2):775-8.

[21] Tearney GJ, Yabushita H, Houser SL, Aretz HT, Jang IK, Schlendorf KH, et al. Quantification of macrophage content in atherosclerotic plaques by optical coherence tomography. Circulation. 2003;107(1):113-9.

[22] Chen BX, Ma FY, Luo W, Ruan JH, Xie WL, Zhao XZ, et al. Neointimal coverage of bare-metal and sirolimus-eluting stents evaluated with optical coherence tomography. Heart. 2008;94(5):566-70.

[23] Finn AV, Joner M, Nakazawa G, Kolodgie F, Newell J, John MC, et al. Pathological correlates of late drug-eluting stent thrombosis: strut coverage as a marker of endo-thelialization. Circulation. 2007;115(18):2435-41.

[24] Joner M, Finn AV, Farb A, Mont EK, Kolodgie FD, Ladich E, et al. Pathology of drug-eluting stents in humans: delayed healing and late thrombotic risk. Journal of the American College of Cardiology. 2006;48(1):193-202.

[25] Gonzalo N, Serruys PW, Okamura T, van Beusekom HM, Garcia-Garcia HM, van So-est G, et al. Optical coherence tomography patterns of stent restenosis. American heart journal. 2009;158(2):284-93.

[26] Tearney GJ, Waxman S, Shishkov M, Vakoc BJ, Suter MJ, Freilich MI, et al. Three-di-mensional coronary artery microscopy by intracoronary optical frequency domain imaging. JACC Cardiovascular imaging. 2008;1(6):752-61.

[27] Liu L, Gardecki JA, Nadkarni SK, Toussaint JD, Yagi Y, Bouma BE, et al. Imaging the subcellular structure of human coronary atherosclerosis using micro-optical coher-ence tomography. Nature medicine. 2011;17(8):1010-4.

Chapter 8

A Noninvasive Alternative to Coronary Angiography: Myocardial Contrast Echocardiography Following Strain Map as a Gate Way to Myocardial Contrast Echocardiography Map

Ri-ichiro Kakihara

Additional information is available at the end of the chapter

1. Introduction

[Background] Segmental left ventricular (LV) wall systolic dysfunction has been considered a significant sign of coronary artery disease (CAD) for many years. However, it is well known that many heart diseases besides CAD cause abnormal LV wall motion. Therefore, it is essential to verify that segmental LV wall systolic dysfunction is due to myocardial ischemia. Although coronary angiography is typically used to determine the clinical significance of CAD, it is also possible to visualize areas of ischemic myocardium noninvasively by echocardiography using microbubble contrast agents. Perfluorobutane microbubbles, consisting of a hydrogenated egg-phosphatidylserine shell encapsulating perfluorobutane gas, offers the advantage of resistance to destruction by ultrasound, thus enabling repeated scans per injection.

[Methods] We used phase-inversion harmonic ultrasonography to assess the ability of perfluorobutane microbubbles to detect ischemic myocardial areas due to coronary artery stenosis in 66 patients who had undergone coronary angiography (CAG). Abnormal LV wall motion was detected by longitudinal strain before CAG. Pre and post-injection images were evaluated from late-diastolic points along the time-intensity curve.

[Results] The injection of perfluorobutane microbubbles caused a significant change in intensity in the left ventricular wall in the AP and SAX views in segments perfused by normal coronary arteries ($p<0.0001$), but not in segments perfused by arteries with significant ($\geq$ 75%) stenosis. Receiver operating characteristic curve analysis showed that an intensity difference ≤ 6.3 dB in the AP view could detect ≥ 75% stenosis with a sensitivity of 98%, specificity of 94% and accuracy of 97%. An intensity difference ≤ 5.1 dB in the SAX view could detect ≥ 75% stenosis with a sensitivity of 97%, specificity of 96% and accuracy of 97%.

[Conclusions] These data indicate that when optimal signal intensity difference parameters have been accurately defined, perfluorobutane microbubbles can be used safely for highly sensitive, specific and accurate visualization of ischemic myocardial areas due to coronary artery stenosis.

2. Background

The ability to prevent, diagnosis and treat cardiac disease has improved over the last two decades due to the remarkable and seemingly exponential advances in imaging technology [1,2,3,4]. Ironically, the surprising increases in computing power and software design now at the physician's disposal have been greatly enhanced by the advent of a relatively uncomplicated and a readily-synthesized molecule, the microbubble. Perfluorobutane microbubbles consist of a macromolecular shell encapsulating a high molecular weight gas [5] and are typically 1 to 10 μ in diameter. Their small size allows them to be introduced safely into the circulatory system where they enhance ultrasonic wave scattering by blood, thereby providing higher contrast to ultrasound images of the left ventricular myocardial wall. Ultrascanners operating at frequencies < 15 MHz oscillate the microbubbles, which results in increased echo contrast. The vibrating microbubbles also emit harmonic signals that can preferentially enhance the signal-to-noise ratio. In addition to their diagnostic advantages, microbubbles also avoid the use of radiation and are generally more economical to use. Microbubble ultrasound technology has been used to image other organs besides the heart (liver, pancreas, breast and kidney, in particular), and can be used to target drug-delivery vehicles to different organs [6]. Basic biomedical researchers are also benefitting from microbubble reagents for delivering macromolecules, such as plasmid DNAs, into cells [7].

Two microbubble contrast agents for cardiac echocardiography, OPTISON™ and Definity™, are approved for use in the United States, SonoVue™ is approved in Europe and China, and Levovist in Japan. But OPTISON™ and Definity™ are used for opacification of the left ventricular cavity and endocardial border definition only. Levovist is used for myocardial contrast echocardiography (MCE). Safety problems occurred initially with each agent, but continuing clinical studies overwhelmingly indicated their efficacy and safety [8,9]. More recently, contrast-enhanced ultrasound (CEUS) has been found safe for pediatric use in subjects as young as two years old [10]. Furthermore, at the recent *16th European Symposium on Ultrasound Contrast Imaging in Rotterdam*, Porter (USA) presented highly compelling evidence that CEUS improved the prediction of patient outcomes when compared with nuclear imaging or non-contrast ultrasound. He also pointed out that contrast imaging avoids subjecting patients to the ionizing radiation inherent in nuclear techniques and suggested that there was significant underutilization of CEUS.

Because of these findings and our own clinical experience, we have persisted in our studies on perfluorobutane microbubbles for coronary artery disease. However, at the present time, this contrast agent has only been approved for hepatic diseases in Japan [11]. Here, we report our experience with the use of perfluorobutane microbubbles to perform MCE in 66 patients who had undergone coronary angiography. Our data showed that perfluorobutane microbubbles markedly and stably enhance visualization of ischemic myocardial areas due to significant coronary artery stenosis and provided superior images compared with Levovist™, but with the caveat that imaging parameters require careful optimization.

3. Materials and Methods

3.1. Patients

Sixty-six patients with a history of coronary angiography (CAG) within the last three months were enrolled in this study, and informed consent was obtained. The study was approved by the clinic's ethics committee. All procedures were performed in accordance with The Code of Ethics of the World Medical Association (Declaration of Helsinki) for experiments involving humans. The following aspects of the consent form were explained to the patients: 1) the advantages, benefits, risks and possible side effects of the procedure to them specifically as well as to patients with coronary artery disease in general, 2) the cost of the procedure according to the regulations of the National Health Service, 3) the approximate time of the procedure, and 4) the clinic staff and specialists that would be present during the procedure. In addition, the approval of the ethics committee required that the procedure be performed by a special team that included the following personnel: Dr. R. Kakihara since he was in charge of the study, the nurses and echocardiographers who had experience with MCE, at least one specialist in the use of Sonazoid™ from Daiichi Sankyo Co. Ltd, and a mechanical engineer and a technical specialist to operate the Vivid 7 Ultrasound System. All 24 patients enrolled had ≥ 75% significant coronary artery stenosis (significant stenosis). Among them, single vessel disease was present in 11 patients, double vessel disease in 9 and triple vessel disease in 4. No subject had a history of previous myocardial infarction. The following patient data were obtained: age, 69.9±11.4 y/o; body weight, 60.5±12.1 kg; body surface area, 1.61±4.3 m²; blood pressure, 128.6±15.3/ 67.7±9.9 mmHg; heart rate, 65.3±9.0 beats/min; LVEF (by angiography), 60.5±4.3%; LDL-cholesterol, 125.6±38.1 mg/dl; and triglyceride, 193.1±134.1 mg/dl. Six patients were treated for diabetes mellitus by oral medication and their average HbA1c was 6.3±1.5%.

3.2. Instrumentation

Phase-inversion harmonic ultrasonography was performed using the Vivid 7 Dimension digital ultrasound system, Version 7.0.3 (General Electric Healthcare, Inc., U.S.A.), and a 1.5/4.0 MHz active-matrix array (AMA) probe. The images were analyzed offline using EchoPAC PC Version 108.1.4. Phase inversion harmonic sonography is two phase-inverted but otherwise identical sonographic pulses are transmitted. Summing the returning echoes in a buffer cancels most of the fundamental and odd harmonic echoes and effectively amplifies the second harmonic. [12]

3.3. The first step

A longitudinal peak systolic strain map (LPSSM) has high diagnostic reliability to detect segmental left ventricular wall abnormalities. [13,14] Thus, an LPSSM was created on any patient with coronary artery disease (CAD) risk factors. When the LPSSM showed abnormal left ventricular segmental wall systolic function, myocardial contrast echocardiography (MCE) was done using Sonazoid™ to confirm whether the dysfunction was due to myocardial ischemia.

3.4. The second step

Materials: Sonazoid™ was obtained from Daiichi Sankyo Co. Ltd. (Tokyo, Japan).

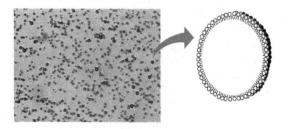

Figure 1. Magnified reconstituted Sonazoid solution. A macromolecular shell is encapsulated by a high molecular weight gas. The microbubbles are very weak and are destroyed easily by usual physical pressure and MI (mechanical index). Sonazoid reconstituted in saline for injection of 2.5mL: Volume concentration: 6.9µL MB/mL Particle size: 2.3~2.9µm (median diameter) Involving gas: Perflubutane (C4F10) Membrane element: Hydrogenated egg phosphatidyl serine (sodium) pH: 5.7~7.0 Osmotic pressure ratio: 0.9~1.1

Any remaining Sonazoid should be stored at room temperature and used within 2 hours.

Because Sonazoid™ microbubbles are susceptible to destruction by physical pressure, 2.5 ml were injected over at least 20 sec, not less than the systemic circulation time under the stress of low dose ATP (0.15 mg/kg/min of Adenosine 5- Triphosphate Disodium) Figure 1, Figure 2, Figure 3, Figure 4.

Measurements: The echocardiographer was blinded to the results of CAG in the patients enrolled. Three apex approach (AP) views and one parasternal short axis (SAX) view were recorded per injection. The instrument settings were as follows: mechanical index (MI), 0.4-0.6 for the AP and 0.22 for the SAX views; frame rate, 21.2; and frequency, 1.5/3.0 MHz. These were selected based on the recommendations of the specialist from Daiichi Sankyo Co. Ltd who had experience with liver imaging. The MI was very low so as not to destroy the microbubbles but high enough to vibrate them. This vibration energy is necessary to create ultrasonic cardiac images. The images taken were clear and of sufficient quality to be analyzed at these settings. The images were acquired from the time-intensity curve in late diastole just before the P wave. Intensity differences before and after Sonazoid™ injection were measured at the same site. The intensity data were automatically shown on the upper right part of the screen. We examined 3 AP views (APLAX: mid-anterior septum & mid-posterior segment; AP2ch: mid-anterior and mid-inferior segment; AP4ch: mid lateral and mid-septal segments) and mid-papillary muscle level SAX views (mid-anterior, mid-lateral, mid-posterior, mid-inferior, mid-septal a mid-anterior septal segments). The segments in the 3 AP views that were perfused by coronary arteries with significant stenosis were designated as Group A and the segments in the SAX views were designated as Group B. The segments in the AP views that were perfused by normal or coronary arteries without significant stenosis were designated as Group C and the segments in the SAX views were designated as Group D. We compared the intensities of all four groups before and after Sonazoidinjection using a paired t-test.

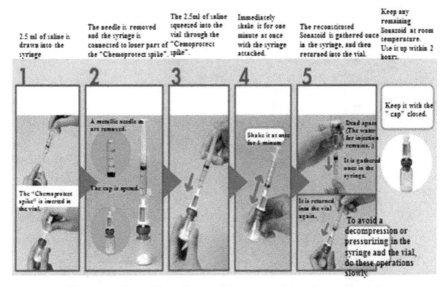

Process of making Sonazoid reconstituted product

Figure 2. Process of making the Sonazoid reconstituted product. The "Chemoprotect spike" is inserted in the vial to keep the pressure in the vial unchanged. Then, 2.5 ml of saline is drawn into the syringe. Then the needle is removed and the syringe is connected to the luer part of the "Chemoprotect spike".Then, 2.5 ml of saline is squeezed into the vial through the "Chemoprotect spike". The solution is shaken for one minute with the syringe attached. The reconstituted Sonazoid is gathered once in the syringe, and then returned into the vial. To avoid decompression or pressurization in the syringe and vial, these procedures should be performed slowly.

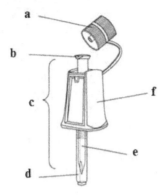

Figure 3. Chemoprotect Spike. This reconstituted Sonazoid production adjustment device consists of a main body, a luer portion, filter housing, spike part, built in liquid filter for drug solution filtration, and an air filter for ventilation. a : Cap, b : Luer portion, c : Spike (Main body), d : Protective cap, e : Protective cap, f : Filter housing, Fluid filter, Air filter

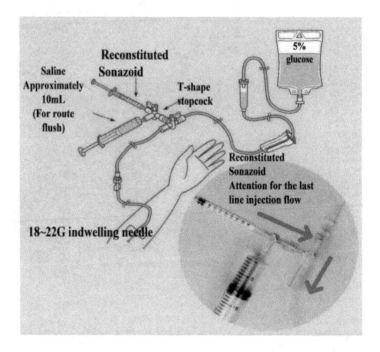

Figure 4. Method and route of injection of reconstituted Sonazoid. Sonazoid (2.5 ml) was injected slowly over 20 seconds. After finishing the injection of Sonazoid, saline (approximately 10 ml) was injected to flush the delivery route

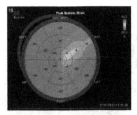

Figure 5. Longitudinal peak systolic strain map. This shows abnormal LV wall motion area, does not show ischemic area. Therefore coronary artery disease is not diagnosis by this map.

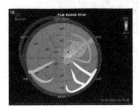

Figure 6. The picture of coronary arteries is superimposed on the strain map. By this method the relation between coronary arteries and the area of abnormal LV wall motion is confirmed.

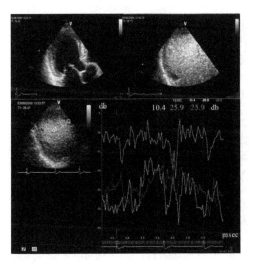

Figure 7. Sonazoid myocardial contrast echocardiography, APLAX views. The patient #7 (see Figure 3 for CAG images) was examined before and after Sonazoid injection. The instrument was set to MI = 0.4. APLAX views before (A) and after (B) Sonazoid. Intensity curves (C). Yellow, LV cavity; red, posterior wall (LCX area); and blue, interventricular septum (LAD #6 area)

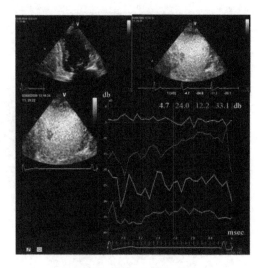

Figure 8. Sonazoid myocardial contrast echocardiography, AP 2-chamber views. The instrument was set to MI = 0.4. AP 2-chamber views before (A) and after (B) Sonazoid injection. Time-intensity curves (C). Yellow, LV cavity; red, inferior wall (RCA area); and blue, anterior wall (LAD area).

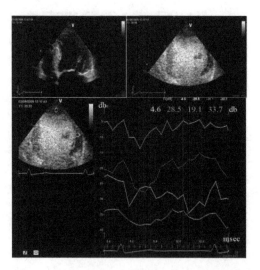

Figure 9. Sonazoid myocardial contrast echocardiography, AP-4 chamber views. The instrument was set to MI = 0.4. AP 4 chamber views before (A) and after (B) Sonazoid injection. Time-intensity curves (C). Yellow, LV cavity; red, interventricular septum (LAD #6 area); blue, lateral wall and apex (LAD #7 area).

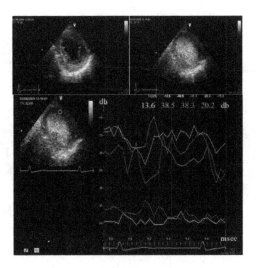

Figure 10. Sonazoid myocardial contrast echocardiography, SAX- pm views. The instrument was set to MI = 0.22. SAXpm views before (A) and after (B, C) Sonazoid injection. Time-intensity curves (D). Yellow, LV cavity; blue, anterior wall; red, lateral wall (both are LAD #7 area); orange, posterior wall; green, inferior wall.

None of the patients experienced adverse affects of this procedure. Each of the 66 patients enrolled in the study had undergone CAG and was diagnosed with significant coronary artery stenosis. Patients were divided into four groups as described above, and myocardial segments perfused by the stenotic and normal vasculatures were examined by ultrasonography before and after Sonazoid administration. The data for one patient (#7) are presented in Figures 5 through Figure 10. Ultrasound images taken before and after Sonazoid administration are shown in 6 Figures, which represent the strain maps and APLAX, AP2ch, AP4ch and SAX-papillary muscle (pm) views, respectively. Figure 5 and Figure 6 show the longitudinal peak systolic strain map and Figure 6 which is superimposed coronary arteries on the map strongly implys this patient experienced no adverse affect and had LAD single vessel disease. Figure 11 shows an angiogram of the left and right coronary arteries. In the left panel, the angiogram (left coronary artery) clearly reveals left anterior descending coronary artery stenosis obstructing 75% of the vessel's normal diameter. Stenotic regions are indicated by the arrows.In contrast, no involvement of the right coronary artery could be discerned.

The data from 100 myocardial segments (16 patients) perfused by normal coronary arteries and from 283 myocardial segments (50 patients) perfused by stenotic coronary arteries in 66 patients with coronary artery disease were grouped into A, B, C and D as designated above and are summarized in Tables 1 and Table 2. Specifically, the intensity difference between A-pre-injection (A-pre) and A–post-injection (A-post) was 1.3 ± 3.5 dB; the intensity difference between B-pre and B-post was 0.9 ± 3.3 dB. The intensity differences in groups A and B were not significant. For C-pre and C-post, the intensities were -33.4 ± 5.1 dB and -22.3 ± 6.8

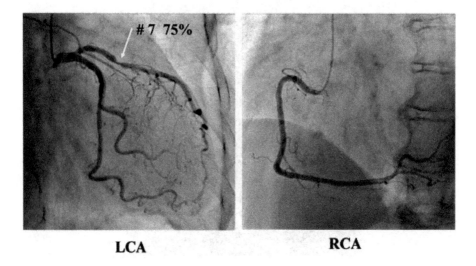

Figure 11. Coronary artery angiography. Left: left coronary artery. Left anterior descending artery had 75% stenosis at #7. Right: Right coronary artery was normal.

dB, respectively; and D-pre and D-post were -36.2 ± 4.8 dB and -22.6 ± 10.7 dB, respectively. The intensity differences in groups C (14.1 ± 5.8 dB) and D (11.5 ± 4.3 dB) were both significant (p < 0.001). By ROC (receiver operating characteristic curve) analysis, intensity differences ≤ 6.3 dB in the AP views could detect ≥ 75% stenosis with a sensitivity of 98%, specificity of 94% and accuracy of 97%. An intensity difference ≤ 5.1 dB in the SAX view could detect ≥ 75% stenosis with a sensitivity of 97%, specificity of 96% and accuracy of 97%. These data indicate the sensitivity, specificity and diagnostic accuracy of MCE using Sonazoid to detect ≥ 75% stenosis.

Stenotic Groups	
Group/View	Intensity difference
A/AP	1.3 ± 3.5 dB (N.S.)
B/SAX	0.9 ± 3.3 dB (N.S)
Normal Groups	
Group/View	Intensity difference
C/AP	14.1 ± 5.8 dB (P < .001)
D/SAX	11.5 ± 4.3 dB (P < .001)

Table 1. Intensity differences before and after Sonazoid administration. A-pre-injection (A-pre) and –post-injection (A-post): 1.3 ± 3.5 dB. B-pre and B-post: 0.9 ± 3.3 dB. The intensity differences for each pair were not significantly different. C-pre and C-post: -33.4 ± 5.1 dB and -22.3 ± 6.8 dB; D-pre and D-post: -36.2 ± 4.8 dB and -22.6 ± 10.7 dB. The differences between C (14.1 ± 5.8 dB) and D (11.5 ± 4.3 dB) were judged significant (P < 0.001)

View	Sensitivity	Specificity	Accuracy
AP (Δ ≤ 6.3 dB)	0.98	0.94	0.97
SAXpm (Δ ≤ 5.1 dB)	0.97	0.96	0.97

Table 2. Sonazoid's detection parameters for coronary artery stenosis. The optimal dB cut-off vales were selected that gave the highest sensitivity and specificity. By ROC, intensity differences ≤ 6.3 dB in AP views detects ≥ 75% stenosis with a sensitivity: 0.98, specificity: 0.94, accuracy: 0.97. In the SAX view an intensity difference ≤ 5.1 dB detects ≥ 75% stenosis with a sensitivity: 0.97, specificity: 0.96, accuracy: 0.97.

The intraobserver reproducibility was determined by imaging the same patients after a four-week interval and then calculating Cohen's kappa (κ= 0.76, p < 0.001). To obtain the four-week interval and then calculating Cohen's kappa (κ= 0.76, p < 0.001). To obtain the interobserver reproducibility, the same images were evaluated by another echocardiographer who was employed at a different medical institute and had no knowledge of the protocol. The interobserver reproducibility was excellent (κ= 0.98, p < 0.001). These two results indicate that the reproducibly of Sonazoid MCE is sufficient for the use of this agent in the clinical setting.

4. Discussion

Remarkable progress has been made over the last decade in medical imaging of the heart and other organs. However, there is still an enormous worldwide mortality and morbidity from coronary artery disease. A major hurdle in overcoming this situation is the inability to make a definite diagnosis of coronary artery stenosis or to screen coronary artery disease easily and inexpensively. Although myocardial ischemia it thought to start from 75% stenosis, patients usually have no symptoms with normal daily activities. When the stenosis is ≥ 90%, patients may become symptomatic with normal daily activities. Presently, CAG is only one diagnostic method, but it is invasive and expensive. Routine preventative cardiac imaging that would be safe (no ionizing radiation or allergenic contrast dyes), highly sensitive, specific and economical would obviously help mitigate this ongoing public health burden.

Echocardiography is one of the areas in which the most exciting advances have been made, and it is especially attractive because it is becoming progressively more miniaturized and can be used in a typical office setting rather than a dedicated imaging center. Current modalities include real-time three-dimensional echocardiography, speckle tracking, contrast echocardiography, intracardiac echocardiography and hand-held echocardiography.

Here, we show that Sonazoid can be successfully used in a local clinical setting and this contrast agent allows the accurate detection of coronary artery stenosis ≥ 75%. This may be accounted for by Sonazoid's resistance to acoustic pressure and its long half-life compared to other microbubble-based contrast agents [15]. Our patients did not experience adverse effects during or after the procedure. This is likely due to Sonazoid's intrinsic nontoxicity, but also by the rapid metabolism of microbubbles via the respiratory system. We compared our results with those of other studies [16, 17] and found similar accuracy for the detection of significant (≥ 75%) coronary artery stenosis. Thus, our data argue for continued investigations into its suitability for MCE and ultimate approval for this purpose, especially in view of the limited number of microbubble-based contrast agents now available to cardiologists. In future studies, it will be of great interest to determine whether Sonazoid is capable of detecting less significant degrees of stenosis.

5. Limitations

The limitations of this method are the same as the limitations of echocardiography. It is difficult to obtain good B-mode images in patients with a thick subcutaneous fatty layer or emphysematous lung. The reliability of MCE to detect ischemia is clearly dependent on the quality of the B-mode images. Another limitation is the process of making Sonazoid™ since the solution is somewhat complex compared with Levovist™. In addition, the detection of ischemic myocardial areas requires the ability to make and read time-intensity graphs. However, we learned to overcome these limitations after four or five subjects.

6. Conclusions

This study showed that Sonazoid™ has good clinical utility and better diagnostic accuracy to detect significant coronary artery stenosis than other contrast agents. This is because the concentration of Sonazoid™ in circulating blood is more stable, and the agent has a longer half-life than other contrast agents.

Comparisons between myocardial regions of affected and normal arteries in these patients before and after Sonazoid™ administration under low-dose ATP stress showed that MCE could detect ≥75% stenosis with a sensitivity of 97%, specificity of 96% and accuracy of 97%. An important factor in achieving these results was the optimization of the MI settings. We believe that these data, taken together with patients not experiencing adverse effects during or after the procedure, provide a compelling argument for extending these studies, with the ultimate goal of providing cardiologists a powerful new tool for routine echocardiography.

The ability of this MCE method to identify various degrees of coronary artery stenosis needs to be confirmed in larger, randomized trials. Although conventional echocardiography cannot detect the extent of myocardial tissue ischemia due to coronary artery stenosis, it can detect LV wall systolic dysfunction due to myocardial ischemia by strain mapping. By applying these two methods, we could develop a new and more accurate diagnostic method. The creation of an MCE map along with a strain map might be used to directly diagnose the severity of coronary artery stenosis and extent of the ischemic myocardial area.

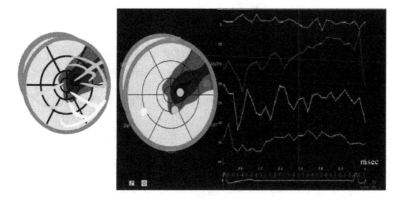

Figure 12. The image of myocardial contrast echocardiography map (MCE Map: left) and the time-intensity curve of the MCE of the patient by MCE MAP.

The extent of the ischemic myocardial area surely play a more leading and important role as an index more than the severity of coronary artery stenosis to decide the indication of coronary artery intervention.

Acknowledgements

The authors heartedly express our thanks to Mr. Yoshio Oonishi (Daiichi Sankyo Co. Ltd, Tokyo, Japan) who kindly provided us with Figures 1, 2, 3 and 4, and also to Mr Kenichiro Morinaga and Mr. Eiji Aoki (SEIKOTEC Co.,Ltd.) who helped me by drawing coronary arteries on strain maps (http://seikotec.com/). In addition I deeply appreciate Mr. Hisashi Koumyou's personal advice to edit this thesis.

Author details

Ri-ichiro Kakihara

Address all correspondence to: ri-ichiro.k@adagio.ocn.ne.jp

Department of Cardiology, Private Kakihara Clinic, Toyohashi, Japan

References

[1] Chelliah RK, Senior R. Contrast echocardiography: an update. Curr Cardiol Rep. 2009; 11(3) 216-224.

[2] Platts D, West C, Boga T, Hamilton-Craig C, Burstow D. Direct visualization of septal perforator coronary arterial blood flow during perflutren microsphere contrast echocardiography. Eur J Echocardiogr. 2009;10(6) 808-810.

[3] Cheng AS, Pegg TJ, Karamitsos TD, Searle N, Jerosch-Herold M, Choudhury RP, Banning AP, Neubauer S, Robson MD, Selvanayagam JB. Cardiovascular magnetic resonance perfusion imaging at 3-tesla for the detection of coronary artery disease: a comparison with 1.5-tesla. J Am Coll Cardiol. 2007; 49(25) 2440-2449.

[4] Schwarz F, Ruzsics B, Schoepf UJ, Bastarrika G, Chiaramida SA, Abro JA, Brothers RL, Vogt S, Schmidt B, Costello P, Zwerner PL. Dual-energy CT of the heart--principles and protocols. Eur J Radiol. 2008;68(3) 423-433.

[5] Schutt EG, Klein DH, Mattrey RM, Riess JG. Injectable microbubbles as contrast agents for diagnostic ultrasound imaging: the key role of perfluorochemicals. Angew Chem Int Ed Engl. 2003;42(28) 3218-3235.

[6] Klibanov AL. Microbubble contrast agents: targeted ultrasound imaging and ultrasound-assisted drug-delivery applications. Invest Radiol. 2006;41(3) 354-362.

[7] Hernot S, Klibanov AL. Microbubbles in ultrasound-triggered drug and gene delivery. Adv Drug Deliv Rev. 2008;60(10) 1153-1166.

[8] Dijkmans PA, Juffermans LJ, van Dijk J, Musters RJ, Spreeuwenberg, Kamp O. Safety and feasibility of real time adenosine myocardial contrast echocardiography with emphasis on induction of arrhythmias: a study in healthy volunteers and patients with stable coronary artery disease. Echocardiography. 2009;26(7) 807-814.

[9] Abdelmoneim SS, Bernier M, Scott CG, Dhoble A, Ness SA, Hagen ME, et al. Safety of contrast agent use during stress echocardiography: a 4-year experience from a single-center cohort study of 26,774 patients. JACC Cardiovasc Imaging. 2009 Sep;2(9): 1048-1056.

[10] McMahon CJ, Ayres NA, Bezold LI, Lewin MB, Alonzo M, Altman CA, et al. Safety and efficacy of intravenous contrast imaging in pediatric echocardiography. Pediatr Cardiol. 2005 26(4) 413-417.

[11] Moriyasu F, Itoh K. Efficacy of perflubutane microbubble-enhanced ultrasound in the characterization and detection of focal liver lesions: phase 3 multicenter clinical trial. Am J Roentgenology. 2009;193(1) 86-95.

[12] Stanton J. Rosenthal, Paul H. Jones, Louis H. Wetzel Phase Inversion Tissue Harmonic Sonographic Imaging: A Clinical Utility Study. Am J Roentgenology. 2001; 176(6) 1393-1398.

[13] Reisner SA, Lysyansky P, AgmonY, Mutlak D, Lessick J, Friedman Z. Global longitudinal strain: a novel index of left ventricular systolic function : J Am Soc Echocardiogr. 2004 June; 17(6) 630-633.

[14] Shimoni S, Gendelman G, Ayzenberg O, Smirin N, Lysyansky P, Edri O, Deutsch L, Caspi A, Friedman Z. Differential Effects of Coronary Artery Stenosis on Myocardial

Function: The Value of Myocardial Strain Analysis for the Detection of Coronary Artery Disease : J Am Soc Echocardiogr. 2011; 24(7) 748-757.

[15] Sontum PC. Physicochemical characteristics of Sonazoid, a new contrast agent for ultrasound imaging. Ultrasound Med Biol. 2008;34(5) 824-833.

[16] I Jucquois, P Nihoyannopoulos, A D'Hondt, V Roelants, A Robert, J Melin, D Glass, and J Vanoverschelde. Comparison of myocardial contrast echocardiography with NC100100 and 99mTc sestamibi SPECT for detection of resting myocardial perfusion abnormalities in patients with previous myocardial infarction. Heart. 2000; 83(5) 518–524.

[17] Binder T, Assayag P, Baer F, Flachskampf F, Kamp O, Nienaber C, Nihoyannopoulos P, Piérard L, Steg G, Vanoverschelde JL, Van der Wouw P, Meland N, Marelli C, Lindvall K. NC100100, a new echo contrast agent for the assessment of myocardial perfusion--safety and comparison with technetium-99m sestamibi single-photon emission computed tomography in a randomized multicenter study. Clin Cardiol. 1999;22(4) 273-282.

Chapter 9

Multidector CT Imaging of Coronary Artery Stent and Coronary Artery Bypass Graft

Bong Gun Song

Additional information is available at the end of the chapter

1. Introduction

Coronary artery stenting has become the most important nonsurgical treatment for coronary artery disease. However, in-stent restenosis occurs at a relatively high rate and this problem has led to the routine use of invasive angiography for assessing stent patency. Although coronary angiography is the clinical gold standard and it is a very effective diagnostic tool for detecting such in-stent restenosis, it's clearly an invasive procedure with its associated morbidity and mortality risks. Therefore, a noninvasive technique for detecting in-stent restenosis would be of great interest and use for following up patients after coronary angioplasty. Multidetector-row CT (MDCT) is being increasingly used for noninvasive coronary artery imaging as it has high diagnostic accuracy for detecting coronary artery stenosis in native, non-stented, coronary arteries. The recently introduced 64-slice CT offers more improved spatial and temporal resolution than does 4 and 16-slice CT and this results in superior visualization of the stent lumen and in-stent restenosis. However, although 64-slice MDCT allows for improved stent visualization, a relevant part (up to 47%) of the stent lumen is still not assessable (Mahnken et al., 2006). The metal of the stents can cause blooming artifacts that prevent the accurate interpretation of a lumen's patency. To improve a stent's visualization, numerous methods have been attempted such as dedicated post-processing or the use of dual-source CT. However, because of its presently limited sensitivity and high radiation exposure, MDCT should not be used as the first-line test to screen for in-stent restenosis in asymptomatic patients. Given its high specificity and negative predictive value, MDCT might be valuable for confirming stent occlusion in symptomatic patients.

Coronary artery bypass graft (CABG) surgery is the standard care in the treatment of advanced coronary artery disease. Notwithstanding the clear benefits of bypass grafting, recurrent chest pain after myocardial revascularization surgery is a common postoperative presentation and the long-term clinical outcome after myocardial revascularization surgery is largely dependent on graft patency and the progression of coronary artery disease. Therefore, assessment of the status of the grafts and graft disease after CABG surgery is an important issue in cardiology. Although conventional coronary angiography is still standard method for assessment of the status of naïve and recipient vessels after CABG surgery, it is an invasive and costly procedure that is not risk-free. Recently, MDCT with retrospective electrocardiographic (ECG) gating has gained rapid acceptance as a diagnostic cardiac imaging modality, allowing assessment of coronary bypass graft patency with high spatial resolution. Initial assessment of bypass grafts was done with single-slice scanners and electron-beam CT. Subsequently, the addition of electrocardiographic (ECG) gating and the improved capabilities available with 4- or 16-slice MDCT scanners for rapid scanning of the area of interest led to promising results in the imaging of bypass grafts (Marano et al., 2005; Ueyama et al., 1999). Recently, the introduction of 64-slice MDCT permitted improved temporal resolution (94 to 200 msec) and spatial resolution (upto submillimeter) and reduction of both cardiac and respiratory motion, leading to improved assessment of graft stenosis and occlusion (Frazier et al., 2005; Lee et al., 2010). Moreover, 3-dimensional (3D) image processing and advanced volumetric visualization techniques now allow radiologists and cardiologists to evaluate coronary grafts in multiple planes using various projections. With the capability of acquiring 3D data volumes along with its tomographic nature, it shares many of the advantages of intravascular ultrasound and thus has the potential to enhance the practice of percutaneous coronary intervention (PCI) in the catheterization laboratory by providing data which was difficult to obtain by invasive coronary angiography (Song et al., 2010; Dikkers et al., 2007; Vembar et al., 2003). MDCT scanners characterized by submillimeter spatial resolution and a temporal resolution of 94 to 200 ms are now available and are increasingly used for cardiac imaging with promising results.

2. Imaging acquisition

2.1. Image protocol

Cardiac CTA technique requires rapid injection of nonionic, iodinated, low-osmolar intravenous contrast. A bolus of 100 to 120 mL nonionic contrast material (high iodine concentration is recommended) is administered intravenously using an automatic injector at a flow rate of 3 to 4 mL/s. A region of interest was placed in the descending aorta by using a preset threshold of 150 HU; a 10-second delay followed before scanning was begun to ensure filling of the distal vessels with contrast material. Axial images are reconstructed in the mid-to-late diastolic phase, using a fraction (percentage; relative delay) of the R-R interval of the cardiac cycle. Images are acquired with a heart rate < 70 beats per minute, if possible, and with breath-holding during mid-inspiration to prevent substantial inflow of unopacified blood into the right atrium, which may result in heterogeneity of contrast. Low heart rates (< 65 beats/min for 16-slice MDCT or < 70 beats/min for 64-slice MDCT) are recommended to obtain high-quality CT scans, and in the absence of contraindications (heart failure, systolic BP < 100 mm Hg, atrioventricular blockade greater than grade I, and referred adverse reaction), beta-blockers can be administered before CT acquisition (Frazier et al., 2005; Marano et al., 2005). Oral or intravenous beta-adrenergic blocking medications, specifically metoprolol (Lopressor; Novartis Pharmaceuticals Corp., East Hanover, NJ), are administered prior to scanning to prevent heart rate variabilityand tachycardia. Retrospective ECG-gated CTA is essential for optimal image acquisition and reconstruction of evenly spaced phases of the cardiac cycle. The images are acquired in a limited field of view with axial images centered on the heart. Using 60% to 80% of the R-R interval, with 0.6-0.75 mm thick images reconstructed in 0.4-0.5 mm increments, axial source images, three-dimensional (3D) volume-rendered images, and multiplanar reformatted (MPR) images are generated.

There are a variety of protocols for image acquisition in the evaluation of patients after CABG surgery. In many respects, the protocol is similar to that for coronary CT angiography (CTA). One important difference is that the scan should be extended superiorly to include the origins of the internal mammary arteries. Scanning is performed with the patient in the supine position, during breath-hold. After placement of the leads for ECG recording on the chest wall and a check of the heart rate, a noncontrast CT scan image is acquired through the entire thorax in order to define the volume of the subsequent CT angiography and to detect associated or unsuspected findings. Hence, MDCT angiography is performed during ECG recording, from the subclavian arteries to the cardiac base; in patients with venous grafts, a smaller scanning volume starting from the lower third of the ascending aorta is usually sufficient. On the contrary, when a right gastroepiploic artery (RGEA) has been used, the scanning volume should include the upper abdomen. Since the left internal mammary artery (LIMA) is the most frequently used graft to the anterior cardiac wall, a right arm venous access is preferable in order to avoid streak artifacts from the left subclavian vein that may hamper a complete evaluation of LIMA course and takeoff. Both 3D volume-rendering and MPR images are used to assess the bypass grafts, proximal and/or distal graft anastomoses, and the cardiac anatomy. In particular, curved multiplanar images with centerlines through the bypass grafts and native coronary arteries are obtained. To correctly assess graft patency and/or the presence of significant stenosis and occlusion, a thorough knowledge of CABG anatomy and its configuration on CTA is important for radiologists and cardiologists. There are 2 types of bypass grafts, arterial and venous. Venous grafts are generally larger in caliber than arterial grafts, and for this reason, jointly to the absence of surgical clips along their course, venous grafts are usually better assessable by noninvasive imaging techniques. In order of frequency of use, graft arteries include the internal mammary arteries (IMAs), radial arteries (RAs), right gastroepiploic artery (RGEA), and inferior epigastric artery. Although arterial grafts have better long-term outcomes, venous grafts, specifically saphenous vein grafts (SVGs), are more readily available. CTA following CABG surgery is done by first assessing the morphology and size of the ascending aorta and the origin of the in situ vessel such as the IMA. Then, graft patency is assessed for homogeneous, contrast-enhanced graft lumen and for regular shape and border of the graft wall. The graft is usually divided into 3 different segments: the origin or proximal anastomosis of the graft, the body of the graft, and the single (or sequential) distal anastomosis. During the CTA evaluation of bypass grafts, the proximal anastomosis is usually better visualized than the distal anastomosis. In cases in which the distal anastomosis is not well evaluated, the bypass graft is usually considered patent as long as contrast is evident within the graft lumen.

2.2. Image noise

The advantages of MDCT are the relatively rapid imaging time and high spatial resolution attributable to the multi-row detector system. Numerous studies dealing with MDCT coronary bypass angiography have reported cardiac and respiratory motion artifacts as the most significant limitations in the reliable assessment of graft patency and stenosis of recipient vessels. It is well known that heart rate greatly influences image quality and stenosis detection. The introduction of 64-slice MDCT scanners, with faster gantry rotation times and shorter breath-hold times, improved diagnostic image quality by reducing cardiac and respiratory motion artifacts. However, optimum performance was observed primarily in patients with heart rates below 70 beats per minute. Even with improved spatial and temporal resolution with 64-slice technology, routine administration of β-blockers is still required. If graft segment image quality is suboptimal due to motion artifacts, a potential remedy is to obtain additional image reconstructions in smaller increments throughout the cardiac cycle. The other limitations of MDCT are the presence of calcification and metal clip artifacts, which make assessment of graft patency difficult, and accurate evaluation of the degree of stenosis impossible. Nevertheless, the thinner slices of 64-slice MDCT give increased temporal resolution, and 3-dimentional reconstructions show consistent detail in every plane. Moreover, bypass grafts are characterized by minor calcification compared to naive vessels, allowing more accurate analysis in most cases. Coronary calcifications and metal clip artifacts still remain a challenging issue with 64-slice cardiac CT despite improvements with the use of sharper image filters, e.g. the B46 Kernel (Siemens Medical Solutions) (Seifarth et al., 2005). The another important limitation is the high radiation dose required for 64-slice MDCT, although electrocardiogram-dependent dose modulation can reduce this by 30%–50%. The minimization of radiation exposure as well as optimization of the diagnostic accuracy in calcified vessels remain the chief goals for future MDCT advances.

2.3. Strategies for reduction of radiation dose and image noise

Current limitations of coronary CTA include image noise and radiation dose. As a result, a number of techniques and strategies have become available on newer CT platforms to enable dose reduction in coronary CT. These include sequential or prospective ECG triggering, reduced tube voltage scanning, and high-pitch helical scanning. Recently, iterative reconstruction (Adaptive Statistical Iterative Reconstruction [ASIR], GE Healthcare) has been introduced as a new reconstruction algorithm (Rajiah et al., 2012; Leipsic et al., 2007; Min et al., 2009). In comparison with filtered back projection (FBP), ASIR reduces image noise (increase contrast-to-noise ratio [CNR]) by iteratively comparing the acquired image to a modeled projection. This reconstruction algorithm is used to help deal with one of the primary issues of dose and tube current reduction for coronary CTA with FBP: increased image noise with decreased tube current. Recently, a high-definition CT (HDCT) scanner, with improved in-plane spatial resolution of 230 μm and the ability to reconstruct images with the use of a novel applied ASIR algorithm, has been developed (Min et al., 2009).

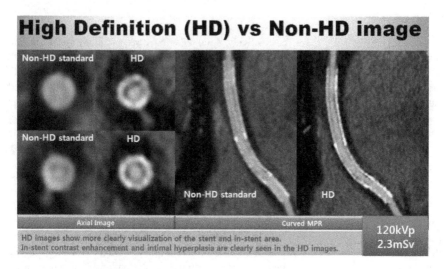

Scheme 1. High definition (HD) versus non-HD CT imagings. HD images show more clearly visualization of the stent and in-stent area.

3. Coronary artery stent imaging with MDCT

Coronary artery stenting is currently the standard practice in nonsurgical myocardial revascularization. However, coronary in-stent restenosis attributable to intimal hyperplasia remains problematic, with an incidence rate of 20% to 30%. The evaluation of stent patency is a major issue in the follow-up after stent placement. It would be desirable to obviate the use of invasive and costly angiography in the evaluation of stent patency. Initial studies using 4-detector coronary CTA for the evaluation of stent patency showed difficulties in imaging small and high-attenuating structures such as coronary stents (Table 1). With 16-detector coronary CTA, coronary artery stent patency has been assessed on the basis of contrast enhancement measurements or pixel count methods. However, stent diameter (≤ 3 mm), strut thickness, and stent material are still a cause of poor lumen visualization. In a study by Gilard et al, 232 stents were evaluated in vivo with 16-detector CT. Lumen interpretability depended on stent diameter: for stents with diameter > 3mm, 81% of lumens were interpretable, compared with 51% for stents with diameter ≤ 3 mm (Gilard et al., 2006). Restenosis detection depended on stent diameter: for stents with diameter > 3 mm, sensitivity and specificity of MDCT were 86% and 100%, respectively. For small stents with diameter ≤ 3 mm, corresponding values were 54% and 100% (Lefebvre et al., 2007; Pugliese et al., 2006). As stated by Kitagawa et al, the importance of metal artifacts and partial volume effect of stents is related to the stent material, the stent diameter and thickness, and the strut design (Kitagawa et al., 2006). In vitro studies comparing 16-slice CT with 4-slice CT showed improvement in lumen visibility, with the same medium smooth body kernel (B30f) for reconstruction (Maintz et al., 2003). The use of a dedicated high spatial resolution reconstruction kernel (sharp kernel or "B46f"), compared with a standard reconstruction kernel (medium-smooth kernel or "B30f"), resulted in a further improvement of the visible stent lumen diameter because, with the B46f-kernel, the stent boundary was depicted more sharply than on the B30f-kernel images. Further, a larger window width to suppress the high attenuation of the stent strut seemed to contribute better delineation and more accurate measurement of the in-stent lumen. In a phantom study, Seifarth et al. showed that the use of 64-slice CT results in superior visualization of the stent lumen and in-stent stenosis, compared with 16-slice CT (Seifarth et al., 2006). In addition to evaluating the in vitro and in vivo performance of 64-slice CT for stent analysis, further developments could focus on the design of stents to reduce artifacts.

Authors	CT technique	Number of Patients	Number of Stents	Stent Caliber (mm)	Criteria for patency	Sensitivity (%)	Specificity (%)
Pump, et al., 2000	Electron beam	202	321	-	Distal runoff	78	98
Knollman, et al., 2004	Electron beam	117	152	2.5- 3.0	Distal runoff	72	60
Maintz, et al., 2003	4-MDCT	29	47	3.0-5.0	Distal runoff	100	100
Ligabue, et al., 2004	4-MDCT	48	72	2.5-4.5	Distal runoff	100	100
Schuijf, et al., 2004	16-MDCT	22	68	2.25-5.0	Distal runoff	78	100
Gilard, et al., 2006	16-MDCT	143	232	2.5-4.5	visualize lumen	100	92

Table 1. Results of studies of the use of MDCT to evaluate coronary stent patency.

3.1. Beam hardening and blooming effect

Metallic struts cause a severe CT artifact known as blooming effect. Blooming effect results from beam hardening and causes the stent struts to appear thicker than they are and, often, to overlap the vessel lumen. As a result the in-stent luminal diameter is underestimated. The energy spectrum of the x-ray beam increases as it passes through a hyperattenuating structure because lower-energy photons are absorbed more rapidly than are higher-energy photons, resulting in the beam being more intense when it reaches the detectors. Calcified spots of vessel wall near or at the outer surface of an implanted stent also contribute to beam hardening, which further erodes the assessability of the stent lumen. Depending on the metal type and the design of the stent, the magnitude of this artifact varies. As a rule, the depiction of stents with the slimmest profile is least affected by blooming artifacts (Lefebvre et al., 2007; Pugliese et al., 2006).

3.2. Partial volume averaging and interpolation

Another obstacle to coronary stent imaging is related to partial volume averaging and interpolation. Inherent in all digital tomographic imaging techniques, partial volume averaging yields a CT number that represents average attenuation of the materials within a voxel. At stent imaging in vessels with a large diameter, such as the aorta or iliac arteries, partial volume averaging effects are present but are limited to the proximity of the vessel wall. In coronary arteries with smaller diameters, the artifacts are of the same magnitude, but a reliable assessment of the lumen is much more problematic. The smaller the stent, the more detrimental the effect of partial volume averaging on the assessability of the in-stent lumen. The thinner detector width on 64-section CT scanners partly solves this problem by reducing the voxel size and thereby the general assessability of the stent lumen (Lefebvre et al., 2007; Pugliese et al., 2006).

3.3. Stent type

The visibility of lumens of different stents varies and this largely depends upon the stent type and the diameter. The blooming effect is more disturbing for smaller coronary stents with thicker struts. Uninterpretable images tend to be obtained for stents with thicker struts and/or a smaller diameter. When the lumen diameter is less than 3mm, the lumen visibility is worse. Regarding the type of stent, the most severe artifacts are found with tantalum, gold or gold-coated stents, or with covered stent grafts as compared with stainless steel stents. Maintz et al. recently evaluated 68 different stents in vitro with using 64-slice MDCT and they created a catalogue of the CT appearance of most of the currently available coronary stents (Maintz et al., 2009). They confirmed that the high variability for stent lumen visibility depended on the stent type, and this was previously reported on with using 4-slice and 16-slice CT. They also concluded that while in vivo studies will be required to verify their results, it can be assumed that a reliable evaluation of lumens of stents in the more advantageous stent types, such as the Radius, Teneo, Symbiot or Flex standard stents, will be possible with using 64-slice MDCT. First-generation drug-eluting stents, which released sirolimus or paclitaxel, were shown to be superior to bare-metal stents and to balloon angioplasty in reducing the magnitude of neointimal proliferation, the incidence of clinical restenosis, and the need for reintervention. Unfortunately, late stent thrombosis (thrombosis that occurs 30 days or more after implantation of the stent) is more likely to occur with drug-eluting stents than with bare-metal stents. The gradual release of the antiproliferative agent effectively inhibits endothelialization of the stent struts, thereby allowing them to continue to serve as a nidus for platelet aggregation and thrombus formation. Second or third-generation drug-eluting stents are designed to provide better stent deployment, safety, and efficacy. They differ from the first-generation stents with respect to the antiproliferative agent, the polymer layer (which acts as a reservoir for controlled drug delivery), and the stent frame. Improvements in stent structure may result in better stent apposition to the vessel wall, improved endothelialization (a thin stent strut elicits less neointimal proliferation and requires less endothelialization to cover the struts completely), and reduced platelet aggregation and thrombus formation, thereby reducing the incidence of stent thrombosis.

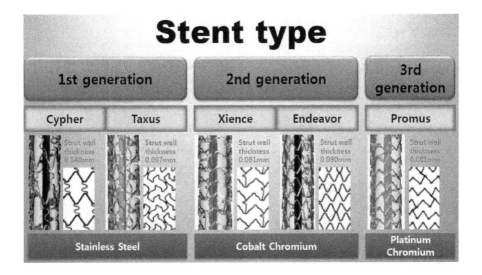

Scheme 2. Detail render of drug-eluting stents. Diverse drug-eluting stents are currently available, differing in the type of metal used, stent design, and drug coating.

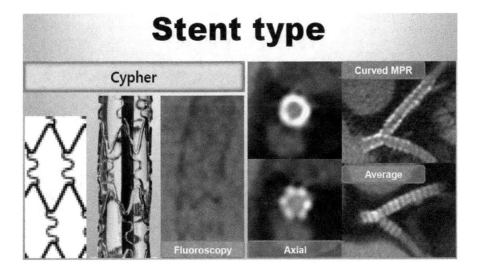

Scheme 3. Type of metal used, stent design, and images of fluoroscopy and 64-slice MDCT of Cypher, first-generation Sirolimus-eluting stent.

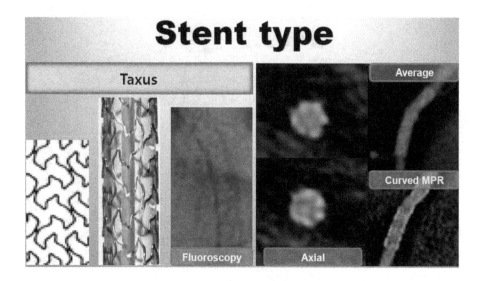

Scheme 4. Type of metal used, stent design, and images of fluoroscopy and 64-slice MDCT of Taxus, first-generation Paclitaxel-eluting stent.

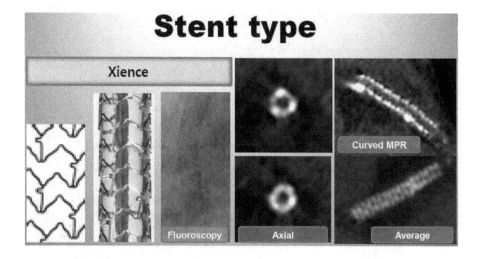

Scheme 5. Type of metal used, stent design, and images of fluoroscopy and 64-slice MDCT of Xience, second-generation Everolimus-eluting stent.

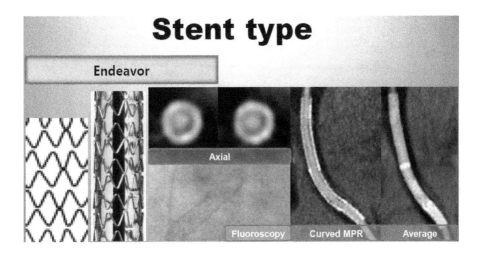

Scheme 6. Type of metal used, stent design, and images of fluoroscopy and 64-slice MDCT of Endeavor, second-generation Zotarolimus-eluting stent.

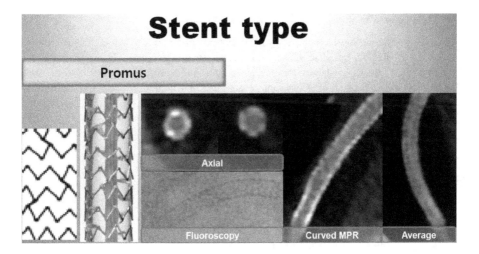

Scheme 7. Type of metal used, stent design, and images of fluoroscopy and 64-slice MDCT of Promus, third-generation Everolimus-eluting stent.

Stent trade name	Metal platform	Coating drug used
Cypher	Stainless steel	Sirolimus (Rapamune)
Endeavor	Cobalt-chromium	Zotarolimus
Taxus	Stainless steel	Paclitaxel (Taxol)
Xience, Promus	Cobalt-chromium	Everolimus (Afinitor)

Table 2. Types of Drug-Eluting Stents Available for Clinical Use

3.4. Optimization of contrast enhancement

Prominent contrast enhancement in the lumen is a prerequisite for robust coronary CT angiography. It is achieved not only by optimizing the contrast material injection parameters (example, using a high-concentration contrast agent and a fast injection rate) but also by accurately synchronizing CT data acquisition with the passage of the contrast agent by means of bolus tracking or a test bolus. Edge-enhancing convolution filters, which may be used for better delineation of stents, have the drawback of producing noisier data sets. If such convolution filter is used, the assessability of in-stent lumen particularly benefits from the presence of high degree of intraluminal contrast enhancement, which somewhat compensates for the kernel-related noise. A high degree of intraluminal enhancement is recommended especially for the investigation of stent patency in vessels that have a small diameter and thus contain less blood (Lefebvre et al., 2007; Pugliese et al., 2006).

3.5. Residual cardiac motion

Residual cardiac motion is of the utmost importance as a cause of vessel non-assessability at MDCT. Residual cardiac motion also plays a role in exacerbating metal-related artifacts such as beam hardening or partial volume averaging effects. The use of high gantry rotation speeds, multisegmental reconstruction techniques, and beta-blockers to lower the heart rate consistently improves the interpretability of MDCT. ECG-based editing techniques allow improvement of image quality for patients with mild irregularities in sinus rhythm, such as premature beats, and for those with bundle-branch block (Lefebvre et al., 2007; Pugliese et al., 2006).

3.6. In-stent lumen evaluation

As mentioned earlier, the direct visualization of the in-stent lumen is important for assessing patency, because collateral vessels may be feeding vessel segment distal to the occluded stent in a retrograde direction. An accurate intraluminal evaluation can best be performed by means of multiplanar reformation of the CT data volume. The stent may be considered to be occluded if the lumen inside the device appears darker than the contrast-enhanced vessel lumen proximal to the stent. Unless severe artifacts affect the CT data set, stent evaluation may proceed beyond a judgment of patency or occlusion. Nonocclusive in-stent neointimal hyperplasia is characterized by the presence of a darker rim between the stent and the contrast-enhanced vessel lumen and is secondary to the healing response to procedurerelated vessel injury. If neointimal hyperplasia exceeds a luminal diameter reduction of 50%, the process is consistent with hemodynamically significant in-stent restenosis. Instent restenosis typically occurs as a localized nonenhancing lesion, often (but not invariably) associated with complex lesion anatomy and discontinuity in lesion coverage. Restenosis may occur either within or adjacent to the stent (within 5 mm of the stent extremities). Edge restenosis might occur because of a decrease in local drug availability, incomplete lesion coverage due to a gap between two stents, procedure-related trauma, or damage to the polymer coating of a stent from calcifications or an overlapping stent.

3.7. Coronary stent fracture

Stent fracture (SF) is an important and potentially serious complication of drug-eluting stents (DES), resulting in thrombosis and in-stent restenosis. Recent reports suggest that the prevalence of fracture ranges between 1.9% and 2.6% (Dimitrios et al., 2011; Lim et al., 2008). SF is probably related to mechanical fatigue of the metallic stent strut, which may be aggravated by highly pulsatile structures such as myocardial bridge, use of long stents or DES unsupported by neointimal tissue. SF may also result from a manufacturing defect. Various factors that have been implicated for a stent fracture include vessel tortuosity, the presence of a right coronary artery lesion, overlapping stents, and the use of a DES such as a sirolimus-eluting stent. In general stent fractures have been reported to be more common when placed in the right coronary artery (RCA) probably due to its curved course, than in the left anterior descending (LAD) or circumflex (LCX) coronary arteries. The type of stent also influences its risk for fracture. The Cypher stent is more prone to fracture as compared to Taxus and Endeavor stents. Overlapping stents are more likely to fracture rather than isolated stents. The presence of stent fracture was classified as grade I to V: I = involving a single-strut fracture; II = 2 or more strut fractures without deformation; III = 2 or more strut fractures with deformation; IV = multiple strut fractures with acquired transection but without gap; and V = multiple strut fractures with acquired transection with gap in the stent body (Nakazawa et al., 2009).

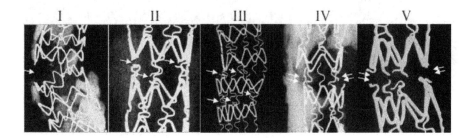

Scheme 8. Classification of stent fracture.

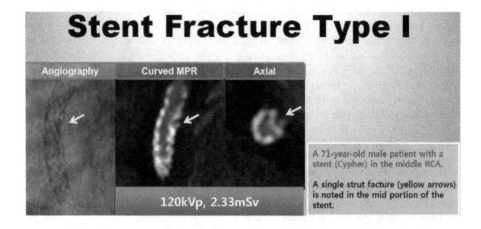

Scheme 9. Images of fluoroscopy and 64-slice MDCT of stent fracture type I. A single strut fracture is seen in the mid portion of the stent in RCA.

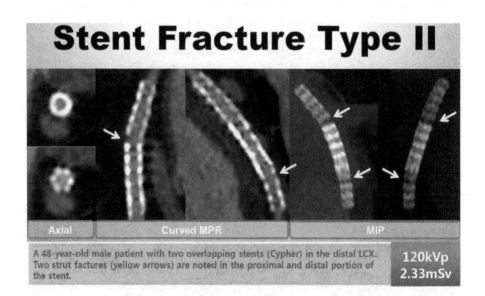

Scheme 10. Images of fluoroscopy and 64-slice MDCT of stent fracture type II. Two strut fractures are seen in the proximal and distal portion of the stent in LCX.

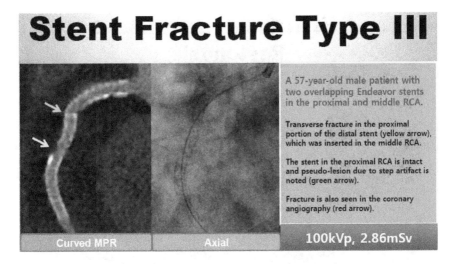

Scheme 11. Images of fluoroscopy and 64-slice MDCT of stent fracture type III. Transverse fracture with deformation is seen in the proximal portion of the stent in middle RCA. The stent in proximal RCA is intact in coronary angiography suggesting pseudo-lesion due to step artifact in MDCT.

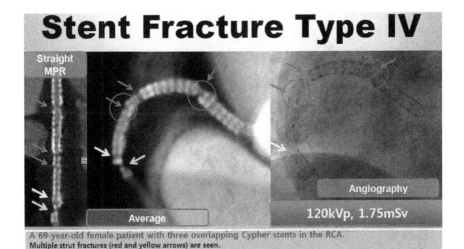

Scheme 12. Images of fluoroscopy and 64-slice MDCT of stent fracture type IV. Multiple strut fractures with acquired transection without gap are seen in the proximal and mid portion of the stent in RCA. The distal portion of the stent is intact in coronary angiography suggesting pseudo-lesion due to step artifact in MDCT.

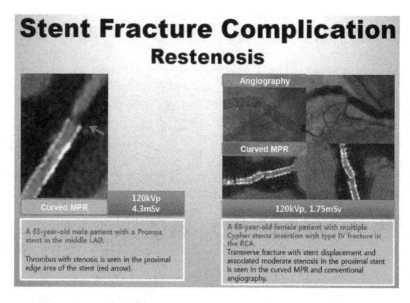

Scheme 13. Images of fluoroscopy and 64-slice MDCT of restenosis due to stent fracture. (Left) Thrombus with stenosis is seen in the proximal edge of the LAD stent. (Right) Transverse fracture with stent displacement and moderate stenosis is seen in the RCA stent.

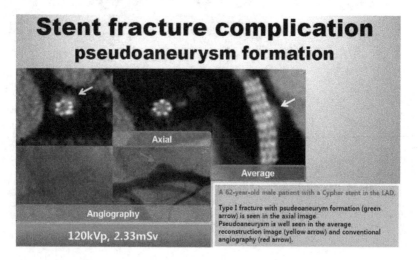

Scheme 14. Images of fluoroscopy and 64-slice MDCT of pseudoaneurysm due to stent fracture. Type I fracture with pseudoaneurysm formation is seen in the LAD stent.

SF has been evaluated mainly by using conventional coronary angiography or fluoroscopy and in selected cases by intravascular ultrasound (IVUS). Recently, MDCT has been found to be more sensitive than conventional coronary angiography in the detection of SF, due to its nearly isotropic multi-planar imaging capabilities, that can depict stents in their long and short axes (Lim et al., 2008; Pang et al., 2009). MDCT imaging on 64-slice scanners provide most of the relevant details required to assess stents on follow-up. In a retrospective evaluation, 64-slice MDCT angiography of 371 patients with 545 stents identified 24 SFs, of which 6 were not detected on conventional angiograms at the initial readings (Lim et al., 2008). An *in vitro* comparison of 64-slice MDCT, conventional cine-angiography, and IVUS revealed that MDCT had high accuracy for the evaluation of coronary SF (Pang et al., 2009). The important features that must be evaluated in all post-stent follow-up include not only the evaluation of in-stent thrombosis, but also features such as stent migration, fracture, buckling, and rarely coronary perforation and aneurysms or pseudoaneurysms (Dimitrios et al., 2011).

4. Coronary artery bypass graft imaging with MDCT

4.1. Coronary bypass graft lumen assessment: Graft patency and stenoses

Coronary bypass graft CT can be performed with 2 different objectives, each with a separate clinical context and goal: the evaluation of graft patency, and the evaluation of graft and anastomotic stenoses. Within the first postoperative month, the main cause of graft failure is thrombosis.75 Graft closure from thrombosis at 1 month is a known complication in 10% to 15% of cases. Coronary bypass graft patency assessment has been shown to be excellent with ECG-gated 4-detector CT, with mean sensibility and specificity for occlusion of 97% and 98%, respectively, in comparison with catheter angiography (Nieman K et al., 2003; Marano R et al., 2004). With 16-detector CT, accuracy is also excellent, with mean sensitivity of 100 % and mean specificity of 99% for detecting bypass graft occlusion, in comparison with catheter angiography (Chiurlia E et al., 2005; Anderson K et al., 2006). Recent studies using 64-slice MDCT have reported sensitivity and specificity values of 95% to 100% and 93% to 100%, respectively, for graft occlusion and high-grade stenosis with > 50% luminal narrowing. Since naïve coronary arteries and coronary grafts are small vessels, 2 to 4 mm in diameter, and are characterized by both complex anatomy and continuous movements, high spatial and temporal resolutions are mandatory to visualize these vessels at MDCT. Vascular clips in the proximity of grafts and their anastomoses, as well as artifacts owing to residual cardiac motion, can be a cause of significant artifacts for the evaluation of graft stenoses.

4.2. Type of arterial or vein graft

4.2.1. Saphenous vein Graft (SVG)

The SVG was first successfully used in a CABG operation by Sabiston in 1962. Both the benefits and limitations of SVG have been well documented in the literature (Bourassa et al., 1985; Campeau et al., 1983). Saphenousveins are fairly simple to access and harvest from the lower extremities, and they are more versatile and widely available than arterial grafts. In addition, during the intra- and perioperative period, saphenous veins are resistant to spasm versus their arterial counterparts. However, the use of SVG is limited by distortion from varicose and sclerotic disease as well as a higher occurrence of intimal hyperplasia and atherosclerotic changes after exposure to systemic blood pressure, resulting in lower patency rates. Graft occlusion can also occur due to vascular damage during harvesting of the saphenous vein. In a large study, the SVG patency was 88% perioperatively, 81% at 1 year, 75% at 5 years, and 50% at greater than or equal to 15 years (Fitzgibbon et al., 1996). The graft attrition rate between 1 and 6 years after CABG surgery is 1% to 2% per year, and between 6 and 10 years is 4% per year. The great saphenous vein is the vein routinely used for CABG surgery. The proximal anastomosis of the venous graft with the ascending aorta is usually performed cranial to the origin of coronary arteries and as distal as the proximal portion of the aortic arch. The SVG can be sutured directly to the anterior portion of the ascending aorta or attached with an anastomotic device, allowing faster, sutureless attachment. The device, called the Symmetry Bypass System aortic connector (St Jude Medical, St Paul, Minn), alters the common appearance of the bypass graft by requiring the aortic connector to be anastomosed perpendicularly to the aorta (Mack et al., 2003; Poston et al., 2004). Recent reports have documented the development of significant stenosis and occlusion in 13.7%-15.5% of vein grafts attached with the aortic connector (Carrel et al., 2003; Wiklund et al., 2002). In order to support the course of the aortovenous anastomosis, the left-sided SVG is connected to the left side of the aorta, stabilizing the graft on top of the main pulmonary artery. A right-sided SVG is attached either to the lower aspect or right side of the ascending aorta, allowing the graft to traverse the right arterio-ventricular groove. SVGs tend to appear as large contrast-filled vessels (Fig.1).

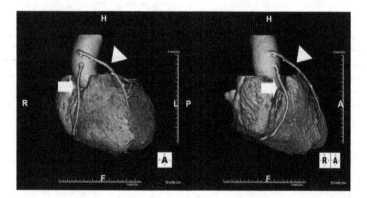

Figure 1. Saphenous vein grafts. Three-dimensional volume-rendered images show the typical appearance of right (arrow) and left (arrowhead) saphenous vein grafts (SVGs) sutured to the anterior aorta. The left SVG is attached to

the mid-portion of left anterior descending (LAD) artery and the right SVG is attached to the distal-portion of right coronary artery (RCA).

An SVG to the right side is attached to the distal right coronary artery (RCA), posterior descending artery (PDA), or distal LAD artery. The distal anastomosis may lie on the phrenic wall of the heart. An SVG to the left side is attached distally to the LAD artery, diagonal artery, left circumflex (LCx) artery, or the obtuse marginal (OM) arteries, by traversing anteriorly and superiorly to the right ventricular outflow tractor main pulmonary artery (Fig. 2, 3, 4).

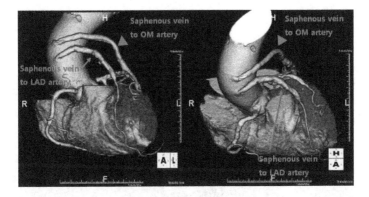

Figure 2. Saphenous vein grafts. Three-dimensional volume-rendered images show the typical appearance of right (arrow) and left (arrowhead) saphenous vein grafts (SVGs) sutured to the anterior aorta. The right SVG is attached to the mid-portion of left anterior descending (LAD) artery and the left SVG is attached to the obtuse marginal (OM) artery.

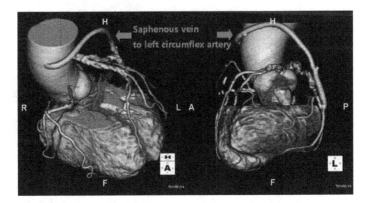

Figure 3. Saphenous vein graft. Three-dimensional volume-rendered images show the left saphenous vein graft (SVG) with its anastomosis with the left circumflex (LCx) artery.

SVG may present a horizontal or slightly oblique course on axial images, especially when the distal anastomosis is placed on the LCx or a diagonal branch to supply the left cardiac wall. In these cases, the graft can be recognized in the fatty tissue of mediastinum, posterior to the sternum and anterior to the RVOT. On occasion, the distal SVG is anastomosed sequentially to greater than or equal to 2 coronary vessels or in the same vessel, using side-to-side and end-to-side anastomoses. The naive vessel distal to the anastamotic site should be assessed and is recognized by its position and smaller caliber compared with the SVG (Fig. 3, 4). Typically, venous grafts are larger than arterial grafts and are not accompanied by surgical clips along their course. Sometimes a circumferential clip can be identified at the site of proximal anastomosis with the ascending aorta (Fig.1).

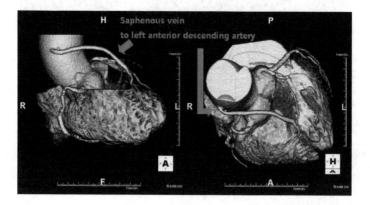

Figure 4. Saphenous vein graft. Three-dimensional volume-rendered images show the left saphenous vein graft (SVG), which is attached to the mid-portion of left anterior descending (LAD) artery.

4.2.2. Internal Mammary Artery (IMA)

The internal mammary artery (IMA) is characterized by unique resistance to atherosclerosis and extremely high long-term patency rates compared with the saphenous vein. The IMA has a nonfenestrated internal elastic laminawithout vaso vasorum inside the vessel wall, which tends to protect against cellular migration and intimal hyperplasia. Moreover, the medial layer of IMA is thin and poor of muscle cells with poor vasoreactivity. In addition, the endothelium produces vasodilator(nitric oxide) and platelet inhibitor (prostacyclin). Glycosaminoglycan and lipid compositions of IMA result in being less atherogenetic in comparison with venous grafts. Therefore, use of the IMA decreases all postoperative cardiac events and mortality, and is associated with a long-term patency rate well >90% at 10 years (Loop et al., 1986; Motwani & Topol, 1998).

4.2.3. Left IMA

The Left IMA (LIMA) is the vessel of choice for the surgical revascularization of the left anterior descending (LAD) artery for its biological and anatomical characteristiscs, being the conduit more proximal to the LAD artery and the easiest to harvest both in median sternotomy and mini-thoracotomy. Due to anatomical proximity to the LAD artery and favorable patency rates, the left IMA (LIMA) is most commonly used as an in situ graft to revascularize the LAD or diagonal artery, supplying the anterior or anterolateral cardiac wall. The LIMA extends from its origin at the subclavian artery and courses through the anterior mediastinum along the right ventricular outflow tract after being separated surgically from its original position in the left parasternalRegion (Fig. 5).

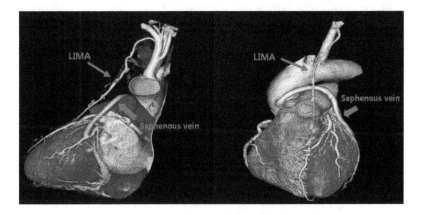

Figure 5. Left internal mammary artery (IMA) graft. Three-dimensional volume-rendered images show the left IMA graft from its origin at the left subclavian artery to its anastomosis with the left anterior descending (LAD) artery. There is also a left saphenous vein graft (SVG), which is attached to the obtuse marginal (OM) artery. Note the smaller diameter of the arterial graft compared with that of the venous graft.

Infrequently, sequential distal anastomoses, with side-to-side and end-to-side anastomoses to the diagonal and LAD arteries, respectively, or involving separate sections of the LAD artery, are performed. On axial images, the LIMA is no longer visible in its usual site, on the left side of the sternum, but courses as a small vessel in the anterior mediastinum along the right ventricle outflow tract (RVOT). Although in most cases LIMA grafts show a single distal anastomosis to the left anterior descending artery (LAD) or a diagonal branch, multiple sequential anastomoses to both the LAD and diagonal branches are sometimes performed. Surgical clips are routinely used to occlude collaterals and to avoid arterial bleeding and can be seen either adjacent to the graft or at the original site of the LIMA. As with other grafts, on CTA, the distal anastamosis is typically most difficult to visualize. Surgical clips are used routinely to occlude branch vessels of the IMA, and metallic artifact may limit assessment in some instances (Fig. 6).

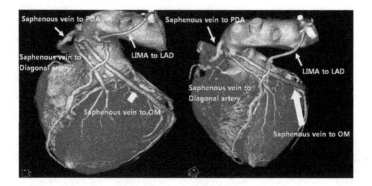

Figure 6. Left internal mammary artery (IMA) graft. Three-dimensional volume-rendered images show the left IMA graft from its origin at the left subclavian artery to its anastomosis with the left anterior descending (LAD) artery. There is also a right saphenous vein graft (SVG) sutured to the anterior aorta with its anastomosis with the posterior descending artery (PDA). The left saphenous vein grafts (SVG) are attached to diagonal artery and the obtuse marginal (OM) artery.

4.2.4. Right IMA

The right IMA (RIMA) is used less frequently than the LIMA. The RIMA may be used in a variety of ways. As an in situ graft, The RIMA remains attached to the right subclavian artery proximally and anastomoses with the target coronary artery distally. However, it is more commonly used as "free" graft from the ascending aorta to the RCA or from the LIMA to the left circumflex artery (LCx) or obtuse marginal (OM) branches. In cases in which both in situ IMAs are necessary for revascularization of the left heart, either the RIMA is connected to the LCx artery or OM branches by extension through the transverse sinus of the pericardium and the LIMA is attached to the LAD artery or the RIMA is attached to the LAD artery and the LIMA is anastomosed to the LCx artery or other side branches (OM or diagnonal branches). Otherwise, the RIMA can be removed from the right subclavian artery and used as a composite or free graft. As a segment of a composite graft to perform an arterial "T" or "Y" graft, the RIMA is anastomosed proximally to LIMA, allowing total arterial revascularization instead of using a venous graft with LIMA. As a free graft, a RIMA is anastomosed to the anterior ascending aorta and used in the same way as an SVG. The CTA appearance of the RIMA is similar to that of the LIMA. As already described for LIMA grafts, surgical clips are used to occlude collaterals. Studies have shown that total arterial myocardial revascularzation has the advantages of decreased recurrent angina and superior patency rates at 1 year when compared with those of conventional coronary artery bypass surgery in which a LIMA graft is coupled with an SVG (Muneretto et al., 2003).

4.2.5. Radial Artery (RA)

The first use of the radial artery (RA) as arterial conduit for coronary revascularization has been de-scribed by Carpentier et al in 1971 (Carpentier et al., 1973). As a muscular artery from the forearm, the RA has a prominent medial layer and elevated vasoreactivity, which results in a lower patency rate than that of IMA grafts (Possati et al., 2003). The RA is usually harvested from the nondominant arm and is used as a third arterial graft, either as a free or composite graft or to avoid using a venous graft in case of unavailability of IMA grafts. The RA is often grafted to supply the left cardiac wall (LCx, OM). On CTA, the caliber of the RA is similar to the IMA, but it typically is visualized coursing from the ascending aorta to the naïve coronary artery (Fig. 7). In the early postoperative period, the RA may be reduced in caliber and may be difficult to identify because of vasospasm. In addition, because the RA is a muscular artery, the number of surgical clips used to close collaterals along the graft is usually higher than with IMA. This may represent a limit for noninvasive assessment of RA grafts with MDCT because of artifacts from surgical clips limiting a full CTA evaluation of an RA graft.

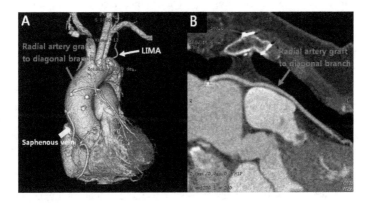

Figure 7. Radial artery (RA) graft. (A) Three-dimensional volume-rendered image shows radial artery graft sutured to the anterior aorta with its anastomosis with diagonal artery. There are also left internal mammary artery (LIMA) graft from its origin at the left subclavian artery to its anastomosis with the left anterior descending (LAD) artery and right saphenous vein graft (SVG), which is attached to the distal right coronary artery (RCA). Note the diameter of the RA is similar to the IMA, but it typically is visualized coursing from the ascending aorta to the diagonal artery. (B) Curved multiplanar reformation image shows patent RA graft within the anterior mediastinum. The full extent of the graft is seen from the ascending aorta to diagonal artery.

4.2.6. Right gastroepiploic artery (RGEA) and inferior epigastric artery (IEA)

The use of right gastroepiploic and inferior epigastric arteries in CABG procedures has been limited because of the need to extend the median sternotomy to expose the abdominal cavity (Buche et al., 1992; Manapat et al., 1994; Pym et al., 1987). Although the use of these arteries increases surgical time and technical difficulty of the surgery, these arteries can be used as a free graft to perform total arterial revascularization. The use of the RGEA was first described by Pym et al in June 1984 (Pym et al., 1987). Although it has been originally used in reoperation, in the absence of other suitable conduits, RGEA is now used as secondary, tertiary, or quaternary arterial conduit to provide all-arterial revascularization. The biological characteristics of RGEA are similar to IMA, but unclear benefits for third or fourth arterial grafts, the increment of surgery time, and the involvement of an additional body cavity are the main drawbacks limiting the widespread use of this conduit. Occasionally, the RGEA is used to supply the inferior cardiac wall and is anastomosed as an in situ graft to the posterior descending artery (PDA). In these cases, the mobilized artery is seen coursing anterior to the liver and through the diaphragm to reach the site of anastomosis. Small clips can be identified at the original site of the RGEA, near the small curvature of stomach. These instances require that the surgical history be conveyed to the radiologist so the CTA protocol can be modified to include the upper abdomen, because the gastroepiploic artery is freed to course anteriorly to the liver and through the diaphragm to reach the target vessel. The inferior epigastric artery (IEA) is an arterial branch of the abdominal wall, arising from the external iliac artery and coursing inside the abdominal rectus muscle. Similar to the radial artery (RA), the IEA has a predominant muscular structure, while the limited length of the vessel with an adequate caliber is a constraint to using this vessel only as a lateral branch of a multiple arterial graft.

4.3. Complication

4.3.1. Graft failure

Bypass graft failures are classified either as early or late following CABG surgery. During the early phase, usually within 1 month after CABG surgery, the most common cause of graft failure is thrombosis from platelet dysfunction at the site of focal endothelial damage during surgical harvesting and anastomosis. Graft closure from thrombosis at 1 month is a recognized complication in 10-15% of cases (Fitzgibbon et al., 1996). Perioperative venous graft failure after off-pump CABG procedures is chiefly determined by the two factors of graft endothelial damage and patient hypercoagulability. Early bypass graft failure can also be due to a malpositioned graft (Ricci et al., 2000). If the graft is too long, it may twist or kink. Technical factors associated with use of an aortic connector may predispose venous grafts to kinking (Traverse et al., 2003). Late-phase venous graft failure is due primarily to progressive changes related to systemic blood pressure exposure. One month after surgery, the venous graft starts to undergo neointimal hyperplasia. Although this process does not produce significant stenosis, it is the foundation for later development of graft atheroma. Beyond 1 year, atherosclerosis is the dominant process, resulting in graft stenosis and occlusion. On the other hand, arterial grafts, specifically IMA graft, are resistant to atheroma development. Late IMA graft failure is more commonly due to progression of atherosclerotic disease in the native coronary artery distal to the graft anastomosis. CTA can delineate multiple findings associated with graft stenosis and occlusion. Calcifiedand noncalcified atherosclerotic plaque is readily identified, and the calculation of the extent of graft narrowing is straightforward. Occlusion can be determined by non-visualization of a vessel which is known to have been used for surgical grafting. In many instances, the most proximal part of an occluded aortocoronary graft fills with contrast, creating a small out-pouching from the ascending aorta, allowing a diagnosis. Acute or chronic graft occlusion can sometimes be differentiated by the diameter of the bypass graft. In chronic occlusion, the diameter is usually reduced from scarring, as compared with acute occlusion in which the diameter is usually enlarged.

4.3.2. Graft vasospasm

Radial artery (RA) grafts are susceptible to vasospasm because the RA is a muscular artery with elevated vasoreactivity. The appearance is similar to fixed graft stenosis, although the luminal narrowing is more extensive in length. Nevertheless, the administration of intraoperative alpha-adrenergic antagonist solution or posteroperative calcium channel blockers can overcome many cases of graft vasospasm postoperatively (Locker et al., 2002; Myers & Fremes, 2003).

4.3.3. Graft aneurysm

There are 2 types of bypass graft aneurysms: true aneurysms and pseudoaneurysms (Dubois & Vandervoort, 2001; Mohara et al., 1998). True aneuryms are usually found 5 to 7 years after CABG surgery and are related to atherosclerotic disease. On the other hand, pseudoaneuryms more commonly occur within 6 months after surgery, although they may also arise several years later. Pseudoaneurysms arise at either proximal or distal anastomotic sites. Pseudoaneurysm cases that are found earlier may be related to infection or tension at the anastomotic site, resulting in suture rupture. In late-onset pseudoaneurysms, similar to true aneurysms, atherosclerotic changes likely played a role. Currently, there is no clear guideline for surgery. Nevertheless, size >2 cm has been a cause for concern (Memon et al., 2003). Graft aneurysms may lead to various complications, including compression and mass effect on adjacent structures, thrombosis and embolization of the bypass graft leading to an acute coronary event, formation of fistula to the right atrium and ventricle, sudden rupture leading to hemothorax, hemopericardium, or death.

4.3.4. Pericardialand pleuraleffusions

Approximately 22%-85% of patients have postoperative pericardial effusions after CABG surgery (Meurin et al., 2004; Pepi et al., 1994). Although pericardial effusions are common, only 0.8%-6% of patients progress to cardiac temponade (Katara et al., 2003). Risk factors include postoperative coagulation abnormality or use of anticoagulation agents that are often related to the use of cardiopulmonary bypass. Nearly all significant pericardial effusions are diagnosed within 5 days postoperatively, peak in 10 days, and resolve within a month (Kuvin et al., 2002). Postoperative pleural effusions are even more numerous after surgery, a prevalence of 89% within 7 days after surgery (Hurlbut et al., 1990; Vargas et al., 1994). These pleural effusions are usually unilateral, small, left-sided, and without clinical significance. Only 1%-4% of CABG surgery patients proceed to develop clinically significant effusions that require thoracentesis (Peng et al., 1992).

4.3.5. Sternal infection

The sternal infection is an important complication of the CABG surgery, with a prevalence of 1% to 20% (Roy, 1998). Three different compartments may be affected: the presternal (cellulitis, sinus tracts, and abscess), sternal (osteomyelitis, and dehiscence), or retrosternal (mediastinitis, hematoma, and abscess) compartments (Li & Fishman, 2003). Risk factors include diabetes mellitus, obesity, current cigarette smoking, and steroid therapy. Surgical risk factors include complexity of surgery, type of bone saw used, type of sternal closure, length of surgical time, blood transfusions, and early reexploration to control hemorrhage. The CTA is important in revealing the extent and depth of infection, which, in turn, will help guide treatment planning. Usually, the preservation of mediastinalfat planes in CTA excludes surgical intervention. On the other hand, obliteration of mediastinalfat planes and diffuse soft tissue infiltration without or with gas collection, or low-density fluid collections within the mediastinum, are concerning for sternal infection. Recently published studies reported a 1-year mortality rate of approximately 22% (Loop et al., 1986; Sarr et al., 1984).

4.3.6. Pulmonary embolism

Clinical diagnosis of deep vein thrombosis and pulmonary embolism may be especially challenging because postoperative atelectasis, pleural effusion, or fluid overload may all contribute to the development of chest pain and dyspnea after CABG surgery. A recent report regarding pulmonary embolism in the post-CABG surgery population showed an overall prevalence of 23% for deep vein thrombosis by 1 week after surgery, with less than 2% of these cases identified clinically (Shammas, 2000).

4.3.7. Incidental findings

Although the intent of CTA after CABG surgery is to assess bypass graft patency and surgical complications, incidental findings are also frequently detected. In a recent study, 13.1% of patients in the immediate postoperative period had unsuspected noncardiac findings, including pulmonary embolism, pulmonary nodules, pneumonia, mucous plugging, and pneumothorax. (Mueller et al., 2007) Therefore, radiologists need to be aware of clinically significant findings with possible life-threatening consequences. 5. Conclusions

Despite image-degrading effects caused by the metallic scaffold of the stent, recent experience with the current generation of 64-section scanners suggests improved assessability of the in-stent lumen with the capability to appreciate more subtle degrees of in-stent neointimal hyperplasia. Knowledge of the different types of artifacts and how they can be compensated for with dedicated postprocessing and appropriate image views and window settings is a prerequisite for reliable depiction of the in-stent lumen and leads to a more robust application of CT findings. In future, the development of biodegradable stents may create optimal conditions for noninvasive post-implantation follow-up with MDCT. In recent years, MDCT with retrospective ECG gating has gained rapid acceptance as a diagnostic cardiac imaging modality, allowing assessment of coronary bypass graft patency with high spatial resolution. This tool could play an important role in patients with recurrence of chest pain or with unclear stress test results after myocardial revascularization surgery. Therefore, it is crucial that cardiologists and radiologists understand CABG anatomy with knowledge of the type and number of bypass grafts used during myocardial revascularization surgery.

Author details

Bong Gun Song

Cardiovascular Imaging Center, Cardiac and Vascular Center, Konkuk University Medical Center, Republic of Korea

References

[1] Achenbach, S.; Moshage, W.; Ropers, D.; Nossen, J. & Bachmann, K. (1997). Noninvasive, three-dimensional visualization of coronary artery bypass grafts by electron beam tomography. *American Journal of Cardiology*, Vol.79, No.7, (Apr 1 1997), pp. 856-861, ISSN 0002-9149

[2] Alexopoulos D.; Xanthopoulou I. (2011). Coronary stent fracture: how frequent it is? Does it matter? *Hellenic J Cardiol*, Vol.52, No.1, pp. 1-5, ISSN 1109-9666

[3] Anders, K.; Baum, U.; Schmid, M.; Ropers, D.; Schmid, A.; Pohle, K.; Daniel, W. G.; Bautz, W. & Achenbach, S. (2006). Coronary artery bypass graft (CABG) patency: assessment with high-resolution submillimeter 16-slice multidetector-row computed tomography (MDCT) versus coronary angiography. *European Journal of Radiology*, Vol.57, No.3, (Mar 2006), pp. 336-344, ISSN 0720-048X

[4] Bourassa, M. G.; Fisher, L. D.; Campeau, L.; Gillespie, M. J.; McConney, M. & Lesperance, J. (1985). Long-term fate of bypass grafts: the Coronary Artery Surgery Study (CASS) and Montreal Heart Institute experiences. *Circulation*, Vol.72, No.6 Pt 2, (Dec 1985), pp. V71-78, ISSN 0009-7322

[5] Buche, M.; Schoevaerdts, J. C.; Louagie, Y.; Schroeder, E.; Marchandise, B.; Chenu, P.; Dion, R.; Verhelst, R.; Deloos, M.; Gonzales, E. & et al. (1992). Use of the inferior epigastric artery for coronary bypass. *Journal of Thoracic and Cardiovascular Surgery*, Vol. 103, No.4, (Apr 1992), pp. 665-670, ISSN 0022-5223

[6] Campeau, L.; Enjalbert, M.; Lesperance, J.; Vaislic, C.; Grondin, C. M. & Bourassa, M. G. (1983). Atherosclerosis and late closure of aortocoronary saphenous vein grafts: sequential angiographic studies at 2 weeks, 1 year, 5 to 7 years, and 10 to 12 years after surgery. *Circulation*, Vol.68, No.3 Pt 2, (Sep 1983), pp. II1-7, ISSN 0009-7322

[7] Carpentier, A.; Guermonprez, J. L.; Deloche, A.; Frechette, C. & DuBost, C. (1973). The aorta-to-coronary radial artery bypass graft. A technique avoiding pathological

changes in grafts. *Annals of Thoracic Surgery*, Vol.16, No.2, (Aug 1973), pp. 111-121, ISSN 0003-4975

[8] Carrel, T. P.; Eckstein, F. S.; Englberger, L.; Windecker, S. & Meier, B. (2003). Pitfalls and key lessons with the symmetry proximal anastomotic device in coronary artery bypass surgery. *Annals of Thoracic Surgery*, Vol.75, No.5, (May 2003), pp. 1434-1436, ISSN 0003-4975

[9] Chiurlia E.; Menozzi M.; Ratti C.; Romagnoli R.; Modena MG. (2005). Follow-up of coronary artery bypass graft patency by multislice computed tomography. *Am J Cardiol*, Vol.95, No.9, pp 1094-1097, ISSN 0002-9149

[10] Dikkers, R.; Willems, T. P.; Tio, R. A.; Anthonio, R. L.; Zijlstra, F. & Oudkerk, M. (2007). The benefit of 64-MDCT prior to invasive coronary angiography in symptomatic post-CABG patients. *International Journal of Cardiovascular Imaging*, Vol.23, No. 3, (Jun 2007), pp. 369-377, ISSN 1569-5794

[11] Dubois, C. L. & Vandervoort, P. M. (2001). Aneurysms and pseudoaneurysms of coronary arteries and saphenous vein coronary artery bypass grafts: a case report and literature review. Acta Cardiologica, Vol.56, No.4, (Aug 2001), pp. 263-267, ISSN 0001-5385

[12] Engelmann, M. G.; von Smekal, A.; Knez, A.; Kurzinger, E.; Huehns, T. Y.; Hofling, B. & Reiser, M. (1997). Accuracy of spiral computed tomography for identifying arterial and venous coronary graft patency. *American Journal of Cardiology*, Vol.80, No.5, (Sep 1 1997), pp. 569-574, ISSN 0002-9149

[13] Fitzgibbon, G. M.; Kafka, H. P.; Leach, A. J.; Keon, W. J.; Hooper, G. D. & Burton, J. R. (1996). Coronary bypass graft fate and patient outcome: angiographic follow-up of 5,065 grafts related to survival and reoperation in 1,388 patients during 25 years. *Journal of the American College of Cardiology*, Vol.28, No.3, (Sep 1996), pp. 616-626, ISSN 0735-1097

[14] Frazier, A. A.; Qureshi, F.; Read, K. M.; Gilkeson, R. C.; Poston, R. S. & White, C. S. (2005). Coronary artery bypass grafts: assessment with multidetector CT in the early and late postoperative settings. *Radiographics*, Vol.25, No.4, (Jul-Aug 2005), pp. 881-896, ISSN 1527-1323

[15] Fullerton, D. A.; St Cyr, J. A.; Fall, S. M. & Whitman, G. J. (1994). Protection of the patent internal mammary artery by-pass graft from subsequent sternotomy. *Journal of Cardiovascular Surgery*, Vol.35, No.6, (Dec), pp. 499-501, ISSN 0021-9509

[16] Gilkeson, R. C.; Markowitz, A. H. & Ciancibello, L. (2003). Multisection CT evaluation of the reoperative cardiac surgery patient. *Radiographics*, Vol.23 Spec No, (Oct 2003), pp. S3-17, ISSN 1527-1323

[17] Gillinov, A. M.; Casselman, F. P.; Lytle, B. W.; Blackstone, E. H.; Parsons, E. M.; Loop, F. D. & Cosgrove, D. M., 3rd (1999). Injury to a patent left internal thoracic artery

graft at coronary reoperation. *Annals of Thoracic Surgery*, Vol.67, No.2, (Feb 1999), pp. 382-386, ISSN 0003-4975

[18] Gilard M, Cornily JC, Pennec PY, Le Gal G, Nonent M, Mansourati J, Blanc JJ, Boschat J. (2006). Assessment of coronary artery stents by 16 slice computed tomography. *Heart*, Vol.92, No.1, (Jan 2006), pp.58-61, ISSN 1468-201X

[19] Hecht, H. S. & Roubin, G. (2007). Usefulness of computed tomographic angiography guided percutaneous coronary intervention. *American Journal of Cardiology*, Vol.99, No.6, (Mar 15 2007), pp. 871-875, ISSN 0002-9149

[20] Hurlbut, D.; Myers, M. L.; Lefcoe, M. & Goldbach, M. (1990). Pleuropulmonary morbidity: internal thoracic artery versus saphenous vein graft. *Annals of Thoracic Surgery*, Vol.50, No.6, (Dec 1990), pp. 959-964, ISSN 0003-4975

[21] Katara, A. N.; Samra, S. S. & Bhandarkar, D. S. (2003). Thoracoscopic window for a post-coronary artery bypass grafting pericardial effusion. *Indian Heart Journal*, Vol.55, No.2, (Mar-Apr 2003), pp. 180-181, ISSN 0019-4832

[22] Kitagawa T.; Fujii T.; Tomohiro Y.; Maeda K.; Kobayashi M.; Kunita E.; Sekiguchi Y. (2006). Noninvasive assessment of coronary stents in patients by 16-slice computed tomography. *Int J Cardiol*, Vol.109, No.2, (Jul 2005), pp. 188-194, ISSN 0167-5273

[23] Kuvin, J. T.; Harati, N. A.; Pandian, N. G.; Bojar, R. M. & Khabbaz, K. R. (2002). Postoperative cardiac tamponade in the modern surgical era. *Annals of Thoracic Surgery*, Vol.74, No.4, (Oct 2002), pp. 1148-1153, ISSN 0003-4975

[24] Lee, R.; Lim, J.; Kaw, G.; Wan, G.; Ng, K. & Ho, K. T. (2010). Comprehensive noninvasive evaluation of bypass grafts and native coronary arteries in patients after coronary bypass surgery: accuracy of 64-slice multidetector computed tomography compared to invasive coronary angiography. *Journal of Cardiovascular Medicine (Hagerstown)*, Vol.11, No.2, (Feb 2010), pp. 81-90, ISSN 1558-2035

[25] Leipsic J.; Labounty TM.; Heilbron B.; Min JK.; Mancini GB.; Lin FY.; Taylor C.; Dunning A.; Earls JP. (2010). Adaptive statistical iterative reconstruction: assessment of image noise and image quality in coronary CT angiography. *AJR Am J Roentgenol*, Vol.195, No.3, pp. 649-54, ISSN 1546-3141

[26] Li, A. E. & Fishman, E. K. (2003). Evaluation of complications after sternotomy using single- and multidetector CT with three-dimensional volume rendering. *AJR. American Journal of Roentgenology*, Vol.181, No.4, (Oct 2003), pp. 1065-1070, ISSN 0361-803X

[27] Lim HB.; Hur G.; Kim SY.; Kim YH.; Kwon SU.; Lee WR.; Cha SJ. (2008). Coronary stent fracture: detection with 64-section multidetector CT angiography in patients and in vitro. *Radiology*, Vol.249, No.3, pp. 810-819, ISSN 1527-1323

[28] Locker, C.; Mohr, R.; Paz, Y.; Lev-Ran, O.; Herz, I.; Uretzky, G. & Shapira, I. (2002). Pretreatment with alpha-adrenergic blockers for prevention of radial artery spasm. *Annals of Thoracic Surgery*, Vol.74, No.4, (Oct 2002), pp. S1368-1370, ISSN 0003-4975

[29] Loop, F. D.; Lytle, B. W.; Cosgrove, D. M.; Stewart, R. W.; Goormastic, M.; Williams, G. W.; Golding, L. A.; Gill, C. C.; Taylor, P. C.; Sheldon, W. C. & et al. (1986). Influence of the internal-mammary-artery graft on 10-year survival and other cardiac events. *New England Journal of Medicine*, Vol.314, No.1, (Jan 1986), pp. 1-6, ISSN 0028-4793

[30] Mack, M. J.; Emery, R. W.; Ley, L. R.; Cole, P. A.; Leonard, A.; Edgerton, J. R.; Dewey, T. M.; Magee, M. J. & Flavin, T. S. (2003). Initial experience with proximal anastomoses performed with a mechanical connector. *Annals of Thoracic Surgery*, Vol.75, No.6, (Jun 2003), pp. 1866-1870; discussion 1870-1871, ISSN 0003-4975

[31] Mahnken AH.; Mühlenbruch G.; Seyfarth T.; Flohr T.; Stanzel S.; Wildberger JE.; Günther RW.; Kuettner A. (2006). 64-slice computed tomography assessment of coronary artery stents: a phantom study. *Acta Radiol*, Vol. 47, No.1, pp. 36-42, ISSN 0284-1851

[32] Maintz D.; Burg MC.; Seifarth H.; Bunck AC.; Ozgün M.; Fischbach R.; Jürgens KU.; Heindel W. (2009). Update on multidetector coronary CT angiography of coronary stents: in vitro evaluation of 29 different stent types with dual-source CT. *Eur Radiol*, Vol.19, No.1, pp. 42-49, ISSN 1432-1084

[33] Maintz D.; Seifarth H.; Flohr T.; Krämer S.; Wichter T.; Heindel W.; Fischbach R. (2003). Improved coronary artery stent visualization and in-stent stenosis detection using 16-slice computed-tomography and dedicated image reconstruction technique. *Invest Radiol*, Vol.38, No.12, pp.790-795, ISSN 0020-9996

[34] Manapat, A. E.; McCarthy, P. M.; Lytle, B. W.; Taylor, P. C.; Loop, F. D.; Stewart, R. W.; Rosenkranz, E. R.; Sapp, S. K.; Miller, D. & Cosgrove, D. M. (1994). Gastroepiploic and inferior epigastric arteries for coronary artery bypass. Early results and evolving applications. *Circulation*, Vol.90, No.5 Pt 2, (Nov 1994), pp. II144-147, ISSN 0009-7322

[35] Marano, R.; Storto, M. L.; Maddestra, N. & Bonomo, L. (2004). Non-invasive assessment of coronary artery bypass graft with retrospectively ECG-gated four-row multidetector spiral computed tomography. *European Radiology*, Vol.14, No.8, (Aug 2004), pp. 1353-1362, ISSN 0938-7994

[36] Marano, R.; Storto, M. L.; Merlino, B.; Maddestra, N.; Di Giammarco, G. & Bonomo, L. (2005). A pictorial review of coronary artery bypass grafts at multidetector row CT. *Chest*, Vol.127, No.4, (Apr 2005), pp. 1371-1377, ISSN 0012-3692

[37] Memon, A. Q.; Huang, R. I.; Marcus, F.; Xavier, L. & Alpert, J. (2003). Saphenous vein graft aneurysm: case report and review. *Cardiology in Review*, Vol.11, No.1, (Jan-Feb 2003), pp. 26-34, ISSN 1061-5377

[38] Meurin, P.; Weber, H.; Renaud, N.; Larrazet, F.; Tabet, J. Y.; Demolis, P. & Ben Driss, A. (2004). Evolution of the postoperative pericardial effusion after day 15: the problem of the late tamponade. *Chest*, Vol.125, No.6, (Jun 2004), pp. 2182-2187, ISSN 0012-3692

[39] Min JK.; Swaminathan RV.; Vass M.; Gallagher S.; Weinsaft JW. (2009). High-definition multidetector computed tomography for evaluation of coronary artery stents: comparison to standard-definition 64-detector row computed tomography. *J Cardiovasc Comput Tomogr*, Vol.3, No.4, (Jul-Aug 2009), pp. 246-251, ISSN 1876-861X

[40] Mohara, J.; Konishi, H.; Kato, M.; Misawa, Y.; Kamisawa, O. & Fuse, K. (1998). Saphenous vein graft pseudoaneurysm rupture after coronary artery bypass grafting. *Annals of Thoracic Surgery*, Vol.65, No.3, (Mar 1998), pp. 831-832, ISSN 0003-4975

[41] Motwani, J. G. & Topol, E. J. (1998). Aortocoronary saphenous vein graft disease: pathogenesis, predisposition, and prevention. *Circulation*, Vol.97, No.9, (Mar 10 1998), pp. 916-931, ISSN 0009-7322

[42] Mueller, J.; Jeudy, J.; Poston, R. & White, C. S. (2007). Cardiac CT angiography after coronary bypass surgery: prevalence of incidental findings. *AJR. American Journal of Roentgenology*, Vol.189, No.2, (Aug 2007), pp. 414-419, ISSN 1546-3141

[43] Muneretto, C.; Bisleri, G.; Negri, A.; Manfredi, J.; Metra, M.; Nodari, S.; Culot, L. & Dei Cas, L. (2003). Total arterial myocardial revascularization with composite grafts improves results of coronary surgery in elderly: a prospective randomized comparison with conventional coronary artery bypass surgery. *Circulation*, Vol.108 Suppl 1, (Sep 2003), pp. II29-33, ISSN 1524-4539

[44] Myers, M. G. & Fremes, S. E. (2003). Prevention of radial artery graft spasm: a survey of Canadian surgical centres. *Canadian Journal of Cardiology*, Vol.19, No.6, (May 2003), pp. 677-681, ISSN 0828-282X

[45] Nakazawa G.; Finn AV.; Vorpahl M.; Ladich E.; Kutys R.; Balazs I.; Kolodgie FD.; Virmani R. (2009). Incidence and predictors of drug-eluting stent fracture in human coronary artery a pathologic analysis. *J Am Coll Cardiol*, Vol.54, No.21, (Nov 2009), pp.1924-1931, ISSN 1558-3597

[46] Nieman K.; Pattynama PM.; Rensing BJ.; Van Geuns RJ.; De Feyter PJ. (2003). Evaluation of patients after coronary artery bypass surgery: CT angiographic assessment of grafts and coronary arteries. *Radiology*, Vol.229, No.3, (Dec 2003), pp.749-756, ISSN 0033-8419

[47] Ohtsuka, T.; Akahane, M.; Ohtomo, K.; Kotsuka, Y. & Takamoto, S. (2000). Three-dimensional computed tomography for reoperative minimally invasive coronary artery bypass. *Annals of Thoracic Surgery*, Vol.70, No.5, (Nov 2000), pp. 1734-1735, ISSN 0003-4975

[48] Pang JH.; Kim D.; Beohar N.; Meyers SN.; Lloyd-Jones D.; Yaghmai V. (2009). Detection of stent fractures: a comparison of 64-slice CT, conventional cine-angiography, and intravascular ultrasonography. *Acad Radiol*, Vol.16, No.4, (Apr 2009), pp.412-417, ISSN 1878-4046

[49] Peng, M. J.; Vargas, F. S.; Cukier, A.; Terra-Filho, M.; Teixeira, L. R. & Light, R. W. (1992). Postoperative pleural changes after coronary revascularization. Comparison

between saphenous vein and internal mammary artery grafting. *Chest*, Vol.101, No.2, (Feb 1992), pp. 327-330, ISSN 0012-3692

[50] Pepi, M.; Muratori, M.; Barbier, P.; Doria, E.; Arena, V.; Berti, M.; Celeste, F.; Guazzi, M. & Tamborini, G. (1994). Pericardial effusion after cardiac surgery: incidence, site, size, and haemodynamic consequences. *British Heart Journal*, Vol.72, No.4, (Oct 1994), pp. 327-331, ISSN 0007-0769

[51] Possati, G.; Gaudino, M.; Prati, F.; Alessandrini, F.; Trani, C.; Glieca, F.; Mazzari, M. A.; Luciani, N. & Schiavoni, G. (2003). Long-term results of the radial artery used for myocardial revascularization. *Circulation*, Vol.108, No.11, (Sep 2003), pp. 1350-1354, ISSN 1524-4539

[52] Poston, R.; White, C.; Read, K.; Gu, J.; Lee, A.; Avari, T. & Griffith, B. (2004). Virchow triad, but not use of an aortic connector device, predicts early graft failure after off-pump coronary bypass. *Heart Surg Forum*, Vol.7, No.5, pp. E428-433, ISSN 1522-6662

[53] Pugliese F.; Cademartiri F.; van Mieghem C.; Meijboom WB.; Malagutti P.; Mollet NR.; Martinoli C.; de Feyter PJ.; Krestin GP. (2006). Multidetector CT for visualization of coronary stents. *Radiographics*, Vol.26, No.3, (May-Jun 2006), pp.887-904,

[54] Pym, J.; Brown, P. M.; Charrette, E. J.; Parker, J. O. & West, R. O. (1987). Gastroepiploic-coronary anastomosis. A viable alternative bypass graft. *Journal of Thoracic and Cardiovascular Surgery*, Vol.94, No.2, (Aug 1987), pp. 256-259, ISSN 0022-5223

[55] Rajiah P.; Schoenhagen P.; Mehta D.; Ivanc T.; Lieber M.; Soufan K.; Desai M.; Flamm SD.; Halliburton S. (2012). Low-dose, wide-detector array thoracic aortic CT angiography using an iterative reconstruction technique results in improved image quality with lower noise and fewer artifacts. *J Cardiovasc Comput Tomogr*, Vol.6, No.3, (May 2012), pp.205-213, ISSN 1876-861X

[56] Ricci, M.; Karamanoukian, H. L.; D'Ancona, G.; Salerno, T. A. & Bergsland, J. (2000). Reoperative "off-pump" circumflex revascularization via left thoracotomy: how to prevent graft kinking. *Annals of Thoracic Surgery*, Vol.70, No.1, (Jul 2000), pp. 309-310, ISSN 0003-4975

[57] Ropers, D.; Pohle, F. K.; Kuettner, A.; Pflederer, T.; Anders, K.; Daniel, W. G.; Bautz, W.; Baum, U. & Achenbach, S. (2006). Diagnostic accuracy of noninvasive coronary angiography in patients after bypass surgery using 64-slice spiral computed tomography with 330-ms gantry rotation. *Circulation*, Vol.114, No.22, (Nov 2006), pp. 2334-2341; quiz 2334, ISSN 1524-4539

[58] Ropers, D.; Ulzheimer, S.; Wenkel, E.; Baum, U.; Giesler, T.; Derlien, H.; Moshage, W.; Bautz, W. A.; Daniel, W. G.; Kalender, W. A. & Achenbach, S. (2001). Investigation of aortocoronary artery bypass grafts by multislice spiral computed tomography with electrocardiographic-gated image reconstruction. *American Journal of Cardiology*, Vol.88, No.7, (Oct 2001), pp. 792-795, ISSN 0002-9149

[59] Roy, M. C. (1998). Surgical-site infections after coronary artery bypass graft surgery: discriminating site-specific risk factors to improve prevention efforts. *Infection Control and Hospital Epidemiology*, Vol.19, No.4, (Apr 1998), pp. 229-233, ISSN 0899-823X

[60] Sarr, M. G.; Gott, V. L. & Townsend, T. R. (1984). Mediastinal infection after cardiac surgery. *Annals of Thoracic Surgery*, Vol.38, No.4, (Oct 1984), pp. 415-423, ISSN 0003-4975

[61] Schlosser, T.; Konorza, T.; Hunold, P.; Kuhl, H.; Schmermund, A. & Barkhausen, J. (2004). Noninvasive visualization of coronary artery bypass grafts using 16-detector row computed tomography. *Journal of the American College of Cardiology*, Vol.44, No.6, (Sep 2004), pp. 1224-1229, ISSN 0735-1097

[62] Seifarth, H.; Raupach, R.; Schaller, S.; Fallenberg, E. M.; Flohr, T.; Heindel, W.; Fischbach, R. & Maintz, D. (2005). Assessment of coronary artery stents using 16-slice MDCT angiography: evaluation of a dedicated reconstruction kernel and a noise reduction filter. *European Radiology*, Vol.15, No.4, (Apr 2005), pp. 721-726, ISSN 0938-7994

[63] Seifarth H.; Ozgün M.; Raupach R.; Flohr T.; Heindel W.; Fischbach R.; Maintz D. (2006). 64- Versus 16-slice CT angiography for coronary artery stent assessment: in vitro experience. *Invest Radiol*, Vol.41, No.1, (Jan 2006), pp.22-27, ISSN 0020-9996

[64] Shammas, N. W. (2000). Pulmonary embolus after coronary artery bypass surgery: a review of the literature. *Clinical Cardiology*, Vol.23, No.9, (Sep 2000), pp. 637-644, ISSN 0160-9289

[65] Song, B. G.; Choi, J. H.; Choi, S. M.; Park, J. H.; Park, Y. H. & Choe, Y. H. (2010). Coronary artery graft dilatation aided by multidetector computed tomography. *Asian Cardiovascular and Thoracic Annals*, Vol.18, No.2, (Feb 2010), pp. 177-179, ISSN 1816-5370

[66] Tochii, M.; Takagi, Y.; Anno, H.; Hoshino, R.; Akita, K.; Kondo, H. & Ando, M. (2010). Accuracy of 64-slice multidetector computed tomography for diseased coronary artery graft detection. *Annals of Thoracic Surgery*, Vol.89, No.6, (Jun 2010), pp. 1906-1911, ISSN 1552-6259

[67] Traverse, J. H.; Mooney, M. R.; Pedersen, W. R.; Madison, J. D.; Flavin, T. F.; Kshettry, V. R.; Henry, T. D.; Eales, F.; Joyce, L. D. & Emery, R. W. (2003). Clinical, angiographic, and interventional follow-up of patients with aortic-saphenous vein graft connectors. *Circulation*, Vol.108, No.4, (Jul 2003), pp. 452-456, ISSN 1524-4539

[68] Ueyama, K.; Ohashi, H.; Tsutsumi, Y.; Kawai, T.; Ueda, T. & Ohnaka, M. (1999). Evaluation of coronary artery bypass grafts using helical scan computed tomography. *Catheterization and Cardiovascular Interventions*, Vol.46, No.3, (Mar 1999), pp. 322-326, ISSN 1522-1946

[69] Vargas, F. S.; Cukier, A.; Hueb, W.; Teixeira, L. R. & Light, R. W. (1994). Relationship between pleural effusion and pericardial involvement after myocardial revascularization. *Chest*, Vol.105, No.6, (Jun 1994), pp. 1748-1752, ISSN 0012-3692

[70] Vembar, M.; Garcia, M. J.; Heuscher, D. J.; Haberl, R.; Matthews, D.; Bohme, G. E. & Greenberg, N. L. (2003). A dynamic approach to identifying desired physiological phases for cardiac imaging using multislice spiral CT. *Medical Physics*, Vol.30, No.7, (Jul 2003), pp. 1683-1693, ISSN 0094-2405

[71] Wiklund, L.; Bugge, M. & Berglin, E. (2002). Angiographic results after the use of a sutureless aortic connector for proximal vein graft anastomoses. *Annals of Thoracic Surgery*, Vol.73, No.6, (Jun 2002), pp. 1993-1994, ISSN 0003-4975

Chapter 10

Nuclear Cardiology — In the Era of the Interventional Cardiology

Branislav Baskot, Igor Ivanov, Dragan Kovacevic,
Slobodan Obradovic, Nenad Ratkovic and
Miodrag Zivkovic

Additional information is available at the end of the chapter

1. Introduction

The strength and breadth of nuclear cardiology lie in its great potential for future creative growth. This growth involves the development of new biologically derived radiopharmaceuticals, avdanced imaging techologies, and a broad/based set of research and clinical aplications involving diagnosis, functional categorization, prognosis, evaluation of therapeutic interventions, and the ability to deal with many of the major investigative issues in contemporary cardiology such as myocardial hibernation, stunning, and viability. The past decade has been caracteriyed by major advances in nuclear cardiology that have greatly enhanced the clinical utility of the various radionuclide techniques used for the assessment of regional myocardial perfusion and regional and global left ventricular function under resting and stress condotions. Despite the emergence of alternative noninvasive techniques for the diagnosis of coronary aretry disease (CAD) and the assessment of prognosis of viability, such as ergo- stress tests, stress echocardiography, the use and application of nuclear cardiology techniques have continued to increase. The establishment of the American Society of Nuclear Cardiology (ASNC) and its educational programs has led to a greater diffusion on nuclear cardiology technology in the community hospital setings and has promoted the emergence and dissemination of imaging and procedural guidelines for nuclear cardiology methods. The establishment of the Journal of Nuclear Cardiology, the official journal of ASNC, allowed a greater number of manuscript to be published in the field [1, 2, 3]

In the few past decade, significant advances have been made in the ability to image the heart with radionuclide tracers under stress and resting conditions in patientse with suspected or known coronary aretry disease (CAD) for the detection of ischemia, determination of prognosis, assessment of myocardial viability, preoperative risk assessment for patients undergoing noncardiac surgery, mand evaluation of the efficacy of revasculariyation in patients undergoing coronary artery bypass surgery or an interventional procedure [1, 2, 3].

For many years, planar imaging and SPECT with 201Tl (201 Talium) constituted the only scintigrafic techniques available for detecting CAD and assessing prognosis in patients undergoing stress perfusion imaging. The major limitation of 201Tl scintigraphy is the high false/positive rate observed in many laboratories, wich is attributed predominantly to image attenuation aretfact and variants of normal that are interpreted as defects consequent to a significant coronary artery stenoses. Although quantification of 201Tl images improves specificity, the false/positive rate remains problematic, particulary in the women and in obese patients. Breast attenuation artifact in women are sometimes difficult to distiguish from perfusion abnormalities secondary to inducible ischemia or myocardial scar.

In recent years, new 99mTc (technetium) labeled perfusion agents have been introduced into clinical practice to enhance the specificity of Single Photon Emission Cumputed Tomography (SPECT) and to provide additional information regarding and global left ventricular systolic function via ECG gating of images [3, 4, 8]. It was immadiately apparent that the quality of images obtained with these 99mTc-labeled radionuclides was superior to that images obtained with 201Tl because of the more favorable psysical characteristic of 99mTc imaging with gamma camera. Perhaps most importantly, 99mTc imaging allows easy gated acqusition, permiting simulateous evaluation of regional systolic thickening, global left ventricular function (LVEF), and myocardial perfusion. One the most significant avdances in myocardial perfusion imaging in the past decade is the development of quantitative SPECT perfusion imaging. Radionuclide imaging is an intrinsically digital technique that is ideally suited for quantification. A number of validated software packages are commercially available for quantification of SPECT myocardial perfusion and function (Auto Quant; Emory Toolbox; 4D/MSPECT; and Wackers Liu CQ), and are carried by the major vendors of nuclear medicine imaging equipment. The basic principles of SPECTR quantification are similar for each of these software packages. Each commercially available package also includes software for computation of LVEF and left ventricular volumes from ECG-gated SPECT images [7, 9, 10, 11].

2. Indications for nuclear cardiology procedures

2.1. Suspected coronary artery disease

CAD is still the single greatest cause of death of men and women in the world, despite a declining total death rate. Using USA data over 459.000 deaths were due to CAD -1 of every deaths. There are aproximatelly 2.2 million hospital discharges with CAD as the diagnosis annually.

The reduction of the morbidity and mortality due to CAD is thus primary importance to physicians and patients. Stress myocardial perfusion imaging (MPI) has emerged as an important noninvasive means of evaluating patients with suspected CAD, with over than 10 millions studies performed in USA annually [1, 2, 16, 17, 18].

Risk factor assessment

The first step in evaluating patients for CAD involves the assessment of the presence of traditional risk factors. Modifiable risks include hypercholesterolemia, hypertension, diabetes mellitus, obesity, tobacco use, and physical inactivity. Nonmodifiable risk factor includes a family history of CAD in first-degree relatives under the age of 60, advanced age, and gender? Once risk factors associated with CAD are evaluated, a patient's risk for having CAD should be assessed. This is often performed by taking symptoms such as a chest pain, age, and gender into account. Symptoms suggestive of CAD, in addition to other risk factors, drive decisions for further testing [2, 12, 17, 18].

A cornerstone of the diagnosis of CAD has been exercise tolerance testing (ETT). The ETT is the safe and easily performed, usually in an office setting. But generally, ETT electrocardiography (ECG) has a sensitivity of 50 to 70%, and a specificity of 60 to 80%.

Thus, the major limitation of the ETT is its diagnostic accuracy for the detection of significant CAD. In patients able to exercise, the diagnostic accuracy of stress myocardial perfusion imaging (MPI) is significantly higher than the ETT alone and provides greater risk stratification for predicting the future cardiac events.

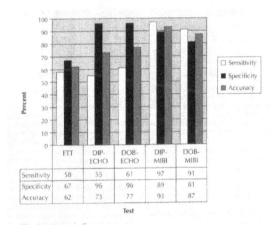

	ETT	DIP-ECHO	DOB-ECHO	DIP-MIBI	DOB-MIBI
Sensitivity	58	55	61	97	91
Specificity	67	96	96	89	81
Accuracy	62	73	77	93	87

(Nuclear cardiology –practical applications)
ETT exercise treadmill test
DIP-ECHO dipyridamole echocardiography
DOB-ECHO dobutamine echocardiography
DIP- MIBI dipyridamole myocardial perfusion imaging with Tc-99m MIBI
DOB-MIBI dobutamine myocardial perfusion imaging with Tc-99m MIBI

Figure 1. Diagnostic accuracy of various tests of CAD

Because of limitation to performed exercise test (patients with medical illness, debilitation, musculoskeletal problems, and the older who can't reach a predicted maximum heart rate) MPI with pharmacologic stress using vasodilators (dipyridamole, and adenosine) or dobutamine can be implemented in such patients. In this moment, it has been estimated that 48% to 50% of all stress MPI is performed with pharmacologic agent. Briefly, dipyridamole and adenosine are potent coronary vasodilators that markedly increase coronary blood flow. This increased flow is less pronounced in arteries that are stenotic (flow restricted) due to atherosclerosis. This causes heterogeneous myocardial perfusion, which can be observed using that follows coronary blood flow as an alternative to vasodilator stress. Dobutamine works by increasing myocardial oxygen demand (through increased heart rate, systolic blood pressure, and myocardial contractility) [5, 6, 7, 8, 9]. As in exercise MPI scintigraphic images obtained at rest compared to those obtained during peak pharmacologic stress to distinguish myocardial ischemia from scar tissue (infarct area).

The diagnostic accuracy of Tc-99m imaging with pharmacologic stress test for angiographically significant CAD has been evaluated in numerous study.

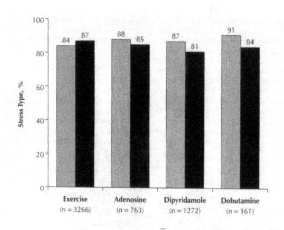

(Nuclear cardiology –practical applications)

Figure 2. Diagnostic accuracy of stress myocardial perfusion imaging.

2.2. Evaluating and determination CULPRIT lesion, in indication for interventional cardiology

One of the most powerfull uses of MPI is the evaluation of the risk for future events in patients with suspected or known CAD. Over the years, MPI has evolved as an essential tool in the evaluation and assessment of patient prior to coronary revascularization. It has a dual role. Prior to coronary angiography, MPI is extremly useful in documeting ischemia and determining the functional impact of single or multiple lesions indentified subsequently. After coronary anatomy is known, and despite some limitations in the setting of multivessel disease, MPI remains the test of choice for indentifying the lesion responsible for the ischemic symptoms, or so colled culprit lesion. That is extremly useful for futher management decisions with respect to percutaneous interventions. In compare, the absence of reversible ischemia in patients with known CAD is an excellent prognostic marker and predicts a low annual event rate.

The current definition of culprit lesion that is zone of ischemia under the coronary stenoses is not quite wright, because that is not definy two pathophysiologic aspects of ischemia; severity and extent. The primary objective of those study was to determinate and localizes culprit lesion by newly introduce parameters SRS (*summary reversible score*) and ISRS (*index of summary reversible score*), under the angiographically detected coronary narrowing ≥75% for the least one coronary artery [2, 6, 9, 11, 15].

In the past two decades, a great body of literature has established the use of nuclear imaging for risk stratification in patients with known or suspected coronary artery disease (CAD). Risk stratification is of crucial importance for the practice of contemporary medicine. Extending the paradigm of noninvasive cardiac testing beyond the detection of disease is especially important, may risk assessment permits patients who are identified as being at a high risk for subsequent cardiac events should receive aggressive management, possibly including cardiac catheterization for potential revascularization procedures that may improve their outcome. CAD is disease with a wide spectrum of severity and extent with outcome, such as nonfatal myocardial infarction (MI) or cardiac death being related to the severity of disease. Clinical trials have shown that patients with severe CAD as left main coronary artery disease, especially those with left ventricular dysfunction, can benefit from coronary artery bypass graft surgery (CABG) with significant reduction in their mortality rate. Whereas patients with single-vessel or with two-vessel disease (without proximal left anterior descending artery involvement) would have improved symptoms of angina following CABG and percutaneous transluminal coronary angioplasty with or without stent implantation, without any effect on their mortality rate.

Coronary angiography, considered the "gold standard" for the diagnosis of CAD, often does not provide information about the physiologic significance of atherosclerotic lesions, especially in borderline lesions. More importantly, it does not provide a clear marker of risk of adverse events, especially in patients with moderate disease severity. Andreas Gruentzig said; *"When coronary angiography founded coronary artery disease, I would like to have diagnostic procedure who will give me functional significance that lesion."* [2, 10, 12, 18].

The presence of normal scintigraphic MPI study at a high level of stress (≥ 85 % of maximum predicted heart rate) or proper pharmacologic stress carries a very benign prognosis, with mortality rate less than 0.5% per year. This finding has been reproduced in many studies. Iskander and Iskandiran, pooling the results of SPECT imaging from more than 12000 patients in 14 studies, demonstrated that the events rate (death/MI) for patients with normal MPI finding is 0.6%, whereas abnormal study carries 7.4% per year event rate, a 12-fold increase [2, 3, 14, 18]..

The current definition of culprit lesion; that is zone of ischemia under the coronary stenoses (what degree? That is not definition. Some autors ofer degree of stenoses ≤ 70 %, some ≤ 75%, even < 80-85%) is not quite wright, because that is not definy two pathophysiologic aspects of ischemia; severity and extent. Iskander and Iskadrian have also shown that defects reversibility is an important predictor of type of cardiac events, whereas reversible perfusion defects are associated with nonfatal MI. This is very important finding, since a reversible defect on MPI imaging is the only available diagnostic tool that can independently predict the risk of nonfatal MI. Therefore, stress perfusion studies should be reported documenting defect severity (mild, moderate, severe), size (small, moderate, large) and reversibility to provide essential risk stratification.[2, 3, 16].

The size and severity of the perfusion abnormality provide powerful prognostic information and has been shown to directly relate to outcome. MPI perfusion imaging and determination of culprit lesion is more predicitble of cardiac events than coronary angiography. As MPI imaging may identify those patients at high risk for subsequent cardiac events, perfusion imaging may be used to help guide further testing and revascularization procedures, and this obviously has important cost-effectiveness ramifications.

The primary objective of this study was to determinate and localizes culprit lesion by newly introduce parameters SRS (*summary reversible score*) and ISRS (*index of summary reversible score*), under the angiographically detected coronary narrowing ≥75% for the least one coronary artery [2].

The rapid rates of technical advances and improved operator expertise have enabled this technique to gain more widespread application. Despite the large number of PTCA-s performed yearly, preprocedure documentation of myocardial ischemia is uncommon, occurring in only 29% of patients.

Myocardial perfusion imaging provides information on the extent and location of myocardial ischemia. The assessment of jeopardized myocardium may be performed and provides a measure of the relative value of PTCA in terms of the amount of jeopardized myocardium. The location of the stenosis may dictate the area at risk: extent and severity of perfusion defects were significantly smaller in patients with proximal compared with distal coronary artery occlusions.

Before revascularization is performed, myocardial perfusion imaging may assist in management decisions by demonstrating the presence of myocardial ischemia, viability and delineating the severity and extent of coronary artery disease. The significance of equivocal lesions may be determined and culprit vessel may be successfully defined by SPECT imaging before angioplasty [2, 3, 10, 18].

The coronary angiography provides information on the anatomical state of the coronary tree and, specifically, on the large epicardial arteries, while perfusion SPECT facilitates the evaluation of the grade of ischemia that a particular stenosis produces. MPI SPECT is of considerable use in the procedural indications of partial revascularization in patients with chronic coronary artery disease (CAD). In these cases the purpose is to detect the coronary stenosis that provokes the ischemia and is termed the "culprit lesion".

The aim of the study Baskot at all. [2] was to determine and localize culprit lesion by MPI in cases of angiographically detected coronary narrowing ≥ 75% of at least one coronary artery.

In the study four hundred and thirty-seven [437] patients were studied. In all of them angiographically detected significant coronary narrowing (≥ 75% luminal stenosis) before PCI. All the patients were submitted to MPI ^{99m}Tc-MIBI, with pharmacologic dipyridamole stress protocol with concomitant low level bicycle exercise 50 W (DipyEX). We measured relative uptake ^{99m}Tc-MIBI for each myocardial segment using short-axis tomogram study. A 5-point scoring system was used to assess the difference between uptake degree in stress and rest studies for the same segment, and we created two indices: Sum reversible score (SRS), Index of sum reversibility score (ISRS). In the results a total 1311 vascular territories (7429 segments) were analyzed before elective percutaneous coronary intervention (ePCI). Overall sensitivity, specificity and accuracy using SRS were 89.7%, 86, 7%, and 88, 2%, with a positive predictive value of 92, 7%. Overall sensitivity, specificity and accuracy using ISRS were 92.8%, 89.1%, and 92.3%, and the positive predictive value was 93.7%. Conclusion this work that is DipyEX MPI with two indices created SRS and ISRS significantly improves sensitivity, specificity and accuracy in the determination and localization of culprit lesion in patients undergoing elective PCI. In this work author defined culprit lesion using two physiological aspects; severity of ischemia and extension zone of ischemia. With quantification of these two parameters of culprit lesion, the author determined patients who underwent ePCI with stent implantation, and who had the best therapy effects with PCI therapy.

Case 1.

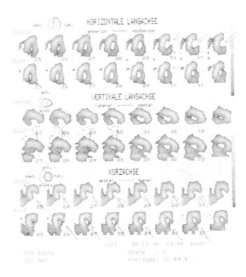

Figure showed culprit lesion in the inferolateral segments in the AdenoEx (up line slices) MPI study

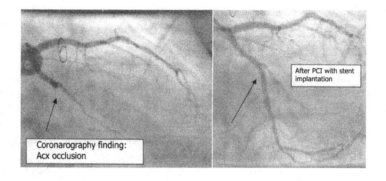

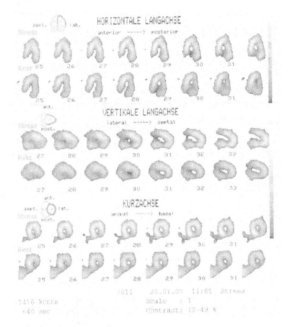

Nearly after elective PCI intervention we performed MPI with normal finding of perfusion

Case 2.

- Patient male 61 year old. St post IM with revascularization 1996 triple ACB (LIMA – LAD; venous graft on the D1 and

- In April 2010 performed SPECT MPI, finding suggested invasive intervention.

- Coronarography finding ;LM 90%, LAD occluded, LIMA graft wide open. Venous graft on the D1 occluded.

- ACx stenoses 90%, OM with tubular stenosis 50 -70%

- RCA dominant, occluded ostial, venous graft occluded okludiran.

- Performed PCI with stent implantation (Tsunami gold 3.5 x 15) on LM and ACX

- After four month MPI control when we founded in stent stenosis.

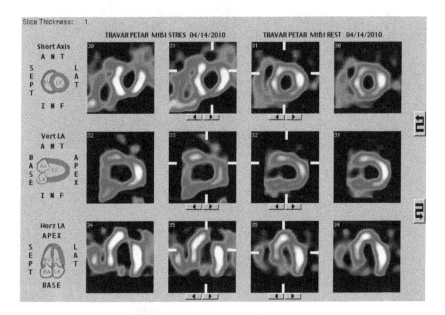

Culprit lesion

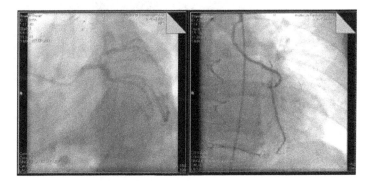

Coronarography finding

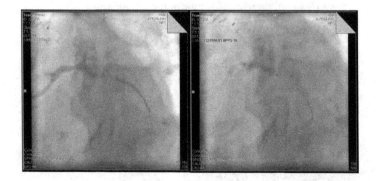

In the same act PCI with stent implantation

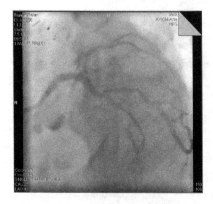

Final effect PCI

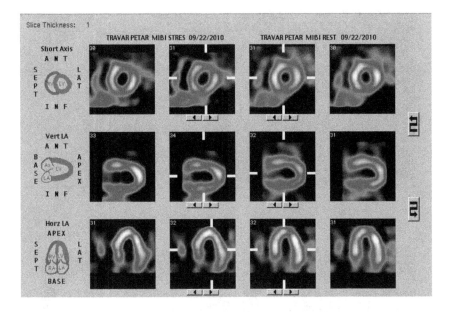

Control MPI after four month after PCI

We finding zone of reversible ischemia in the same area, suggest restenosis

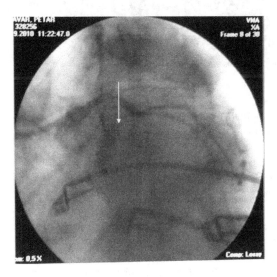

Control Coronarography - fidning in stent stenonis

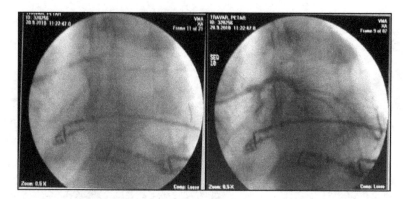

Re PCI with stent implantation

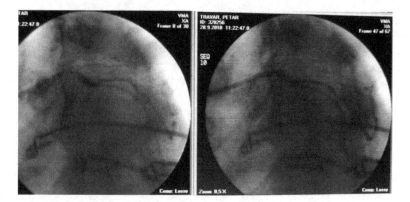

Final effect

Conversely, patients with high-risk scans may benefit from an early invasive strategy with a view toward revascularization depending on coronary anatomical finding. A substantial number of patients undergoing SPECT perfusion imaging will have mild ischemia without a multi-vessel disease scan pattern. If patients with mild ischemia have good exercise tolerance, they should be considered as candidates for intense medical therapy with follow-up exercise SPECT imaging possibly at 1 year. Unpublished data from the Clinical Outcomes Utilizing Revascularization and Aggressive Drug Evaluations (COURAGE) trial seem to indicate that many ischemic defects may markedly improve with aggressive lowering of abnormal lipids an the other pharmacological interventions. Hachamovitch and colleagues reported patients with the mildly abnormal scan had a 0.8% annual cardiac death rate compared with 0.9% for those who underwent revascularization. The death rate in medically treated patients who had moderately abnormal scans was 2.3% versus 1.1% for such patients undergoing revascularization. Finally, patients with a severely abnormal scan treated medically had an annual cardiac death rate of 4.6% versus 1.3% for such patients who were revascularized. In the second study, these investigators showed that medically treated patients who had greater than 20% of the total myocardium rendered ischemic had higher annual cardiac death rate (6.7%) compared with 2.0% for patients with this degree of extensive ischemia who underwent revascularization. For patients with 10% or less of the total myocardium rendered ischemic, there was no difference in outcome between medical therapy and revascularization.

Exercise myocardial perfusion imaging is a valuable adjunct for separating high to low risk patients who present symptoms consistent with stable CAD, or in patients who have known disease and in whom further prognostication is warranted. Multiple high-risk nuclear imaging variables can be identified, and the greater the extent of exercise/induced ischemia, the greater the risk of cardiac events. Adjunctive variables, such as transient ischemic cavity dilatation and functional assessment with evaluation of regional wall thickening or wall motion and left ventricular ejection fraction greatly assist in the risk stratification process [1, 3, 16, 18].

Nuclear cardiology is uniquely placed to address all the major determinants of prognosis in CAD can be assessed by measurements of stress-induced perfusion or function. These measurements include the amount of infarcted myocardium, the amount of jeopardized myocardium (supplied by vessels with hemodynamically significant stenosis), and the degree of jeopardy (tightness of the individual coronary stenosis). Recent evidence in large patient cohorts has revealed that factor estimating the extent of left ventricular dysfunction (left ventricular ejection fraction, extent of infarcted myocardium, transient ischemic dilatation of the left ventricle and increasing lung uptake) are excellent predictors of cardiac mortality. However, measurements of inducible ischemia are the best predictors of the development of acute coronary syndromes. Several reports have shown that nuclear testing yields incremental prognostic value over clinical information with respect to cardiac death, or the combination of cardiac death and nonfatal myocardial infarction as isolated endpoints. Now it is possible to tailor therapeutic decision making for an individual patient based upon combination of clinical factors and nuclear scan results. Patients with severe perfusion abnormalities on their stress image may have a five- to ten-fold higher likelihood of cardiac death versus patient with a normal myocardial perfusion SPECT. If the defects perfusion determined as a culprit lesion, invasive therapy (PCI) is an optimized outcome for that patient [2, 12, 13, 15].

The explosion of PTCA and stent placement in patients with single or multi-vessel disease has created a necessity for early detection of restenosis. A number of clinical studies have documented the usefulness of stress MPI for identifying restenosis in patients after PCI. One point of controversy is the optimal time to performing SPECT imaging after coronary intervention. Although current consensus in to obtain an exercise MPI study 4 to 6 weeks post intervention, whenever indicated, the proper timing for use of MPI remains to be determined. Based on existing knowledge about the timing interval of subacute thrombosis (< 4 weeks) and in-stent restenosis (3-6 month), we purpose the algorithm as a guide for the management of patients with known CAD after PCI [2, 15, 16, 18].

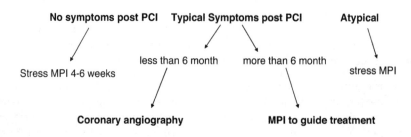

Figure 3. Recommendation for the diagnostic treatment after PCI.

Asymptomatic patients may be considered for stress MPI 4 to 6 weeks post intervention in order to assess the functional results of PCI and established a new baseline. Subsets of patients that benefit from this approach include those at high risk post PCI (patients with decreased LV function, proximal left anterior descending artery disease, previous sudden death, diabetes mellitus, hazardous occupations, and suboptimal PCI results). Stress MPI is also recommended in patients who develop atypical symptoms after PCI and there is necessity to assess whether these symptoms represent ischemia. Patient with symptoms typical of ischemia < 6 months post intervention should proceed with coronary angiography as a first step, unless contraindicated. If angina occurs later (> 6 months post PCI), stress/pharmacologic MPI can be used to assess degree and area of ischemia, since progression of native coronary disease rather than in-stent restenosis is more likely.

Incremental prognostic value of MPI; Because nuclear test are expensive the cost-effectiveness of these tests should demonstrate incremental prognostic information that cannot be derived from less expensive modalities such as clinical patient history and risks factors, standard ECG, and exercise ECG.

The combination clinical and exercise MPI variables provided greater prognostic information than the combination of clinical and angiographic data. Iskandrian et al showed that in medically treated patients with CAD, exercise SPECT imaging provided independent and incremental prognostic information even when catheterization data are available. The extent of perfusion abnormality was the single best predictor of prognosis. MPI added incremental prognostic information and risk-stratified patient even after clinical and exercise information were known. The incremental prognostic information about prognosis and need for coronary angiography provided by MPI has additionally been demonstrated for specific patients subsets: women, patient following coronary angioplasty or CABG, after MI, and with unstable angina. Hachamovitch et al demonstrated the use of MPI to yield incremental prognostic information toward the identification of cardiac death. Patient with a mildly abnormal scan after exercise stress are at low risk for cardiac death, but intermediate risk for nonfatal MI. A noninvasive strategy of optimizing medical therapy in this patient subgroup may result in significant cost saving when compared with invasive management strategy [1, 2, 3, 12, 18].

The prognostic efficacy of MPI is well established. Subsequent data have demonstrated in various patient subsets that nuclear tests add significant and incremental predictive value to less expensive clinical and exercise testing data. Angiographic data obtained from more expensive cardiac catheterization procedures add little or no significant incremental prognostic value when added to the results of MPI.

The introduction of new drugs and interventional devices to treat CAD, coupled with the arrival of manage care, has led to era of cost-containment within the practice of cardiology. Stress MPI is increasingly seen as a gatekeeper for more costly diagnosis and interventional procedures. Steingart et al evaluated 378 patients with a full range of pretest probabilities for CAD, and demonstrated that the results of MPI significantly reduced referring physicians' likelihood of recommending cardiac catheterization, on average by 49%.

Under managed care health systems that operate under cost-containment and capitation, MPI will continue to impact significantly on the decision to perform cardiac catheterization and to refer patients for coronary revascurization. Recommendations for invasive and interventional procedures are often coupled with an appropriate understanding of the prognostic value of MPI. Patients with the normal stress radionuclide study do not generally require referral for additional procedures, even when the likelihood of underlying CAD is high, as based on clinical and stress ECG data. The need for cardiac catheterization and coronary revascularization rates should be based on the degree of abnormality as detected by MPI. Thus, there is an increasing role of MPI to play an important gatekeeper function in the current era of managed care and emphasis on cost-containment [2, 3, 8, 12, 18].

Stress MPI has became a central guide in decision making with regard to CAD patients. Stress MPI is commonly used either before consideration of coronary revascularization or after its performance, to optimize decision making for CAD patients. Stress MPI is also used after myocardial revascularization procedures, to evaluate therapeutic efficacy; following the stabilization of acute ischemic syndromes; to determine subsequent risk; and before the performance of elective non-cardiac surgery, to identify the high-risk subsets of CAD patients who will require coronary revascularization prior to elective surgery.

After all, MPI has became an important instrument in defining cardiac risk and in identifying patients who are most likely to benefit from additional invasive diagnostic testing and potential coronary revascularization. MPI demonstrated significant incremental prognostic

3. Heart failure — New approach of therapy and diagnostic evaluation of therapy effect[1]

Heart failure (HF) is becoming the main clinical challenge in cardiology in the twenty - first century and is associated with high morbidity and mortality. Heart failure is the third most

---

1 Zivkovic Miodrag, Baskot Branislav

prevalent cardiovascular disease in the United States. An estimated 5 million people in the USA have heart failure, and the prevalence of the condition increase to 10 million by 2040, according to prediction. The prevalence of heart failure increase with age from less than 1% in the 20 – 30-year-old age group to over 20% in people age 80 years and older. The diagnostic and therapeutic costs involved are estimated to have exceeded $34 billion in only one year. Despite advances in therapies, the long-term prognosis from patients with heart failure remain poor; 80% of men and 70% of women greater than 65 years of age with heart failure die within 8 years [1, 2, 19, 20, 21].

3.1. What we need for good and quality therapy

The underllying etiology of HF needs to be determined; most patients have CAD (approximately 70% - 80%). Nuclear imaging can help in the differentiation between patients with ischemic and non-ischemic HF. In patients with ischemic cardiomiopathy, the precise coronary anatomy is also needed to determinate if revascularization needs to be considered. At present, invasive angiography is performed to obtain the coronary anatomy, but multi-slice CT (MSCT) may also provide this information. The presence of ischemia and viability needs to be determined to decide further if revascularization is indicated.

Nuclear imaging is considered the first choice technique for assessment of ischemia and viability; booth single-photon emission CT (SPECT), and positron emission tomography (PET) can provide this information.

Nuclear imaging can provide some indirect evidence in the differentiation between ischemic and non-ischemic HF. With stress,-rest SPECT study, reversible defects indicate ischemia and fixed defects of perfusion indicates scar tissue; booth this findings are markers of coronary artery disease. Moreover, lot of studies with nuclear perfusion imaging demonstrated that patients with ischemic HF had extensive and diffuse perfusion defects, whereas tracer uptake (myocardial perfusion) was mostly homogeneous (ischemic) in patients with non-ischemic HF.

Similarly, PET studies also demonstrated that patients with non-ischemic HF had more homogeneous tracer uptake, whereas patients with ischemic HF had areas of severely reduced uptake (reflecting scar formation). Accordingly, nuclear imaging can help in the differentiation between ischemic and non-ischemic cardiomyopathy, but for the diagnosis of underlying coronary artery disease, visualization of the coronary artery is needed. Invasive angiography is the technique of choice, but recently MSCT has been introduced for noninvasive angiography. With 64-slice MSCT and dual-source slice MSCT, we obtained more consistent image quality with improve visualization of the coronary artery tree. In the presence of a flow-limiting stenosis, resting myocardial is preserved, but once an increased myocardial oxygen demand occurs, a perfusion demand-supply mismatch follows, resulting in myocardial ischemia. Then, a sequence of events is initiated, which is referred to as the "ischemic cascade". Perfusion abnormalities occur at an early stage, whereas diastolic and systolic left ventricular dysfunction occur later. Accordingly, such techniques as nuclear imaging that defect perfusion abnormalities should have a high sensitivity for detection of ischemia, because these abnormalities occur early in the cascade [19, 20, 21].

In the heart failure patients, the combination between the coronary anatomy and the presence of ischemia in the territories of the stenotic vessels determines the need for revascularization. In the absence of ischemia, the presence of viability needs to evaluation.

Another nuclear study performed in the evaluating of therapy effects in HF, is radionuclide angiography (RNV). That is the most reproducible, accurate, and simple method for noninvasively assessing left ventricular ejection fraction (LVEF). RNV are now most often used for serial assessment of LVEF in patients who undergo chemotherapy, assessment of global regional wall motion in patients with recent or old myocardial infarction, and in patients with congestive heart failure. In the patients with heart failure, evaluation of left ventricular systolic function is essential to plan management and determine prognosis. At the present time most RNV are acquired by multiple – view planar image technique. In this moment SPECT RNV is not routinely performed in most nuclear cardiology laboratories. The greatest attraction of SPECT RNV is the ability to evaluate cardiac chambers and regional wall motion without overlap of other structures. LVEF may be calculated based on count changes from either a conventional planar image (*best septal*) or from SPECT RNV.

In the pilot study Zivkovic, Baskot at all. We introduced new therapy, hyperbaric oxygenation (HBO) and erythropoietin (EPO) in the treatment of heart failure. The aim of this study is to show positive therapeutic effects of synergistic applications of HBO as a strong generator of regenerator activities in human tissues, and recombinant EPO as a general growth factor, in the treatment HF ischemic and non-ischemic origin [19, 20, 21].

HBO is medical procedure of breathing the 100% oxygen under pressures higher than atmospheric pressure is and it carries out into hyperbaric chambers. Contemporary, HBO changes the rheological blood characteristic, recovers the function of blood vessels endothelium and it has good antiaggregation effects. The oxygen's pharmacokinetic and neo-angiogenesis effects and its effect on oxygen-dependent reactions inside the mitochondria's and homeopathy effect on the other organs are the reasons to use HBO in the treatment of HF. Nuclear imaging by SPECT imaging in the evaluation between ischemic and non-ischemic HF we performed, and followed with quantification per segments before and after therapy in the evaluation positive therapeutic effect. We also performed RNV like gold standard in the evaluation global and regional LVEF before and after the therapy. In the pilot study with 18 patients, we had recovery perfusion in all patients with non-ischemic HF. Before therapy we finding with RNV average measured LVEF was 23.4%. After treatment LVEF measured average 34, 3%. The results was increase by 10, 9% (from 5% to 20% measured individually).

Conclusion of this pilot study was that diagnostic information finding by nuclear cardiology (perfusion and function) suggested significantly positive therapy effects HBO and Erythropoietin in the therapy of heart failure ischemic and non-ischemic origin.

Case report 1. Patient female with multi vessel disease by coronarography

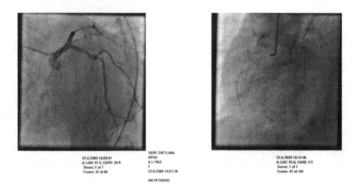

SPECT with DipyEX (dipyridamole = concomitant low level exercise 50W) performed and evaluated before and after HBO + EPO therapy

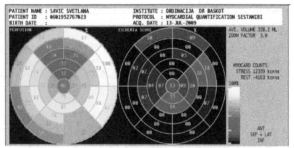

quantification of perfusion by Stierner
- segments quantification 07.13.2009

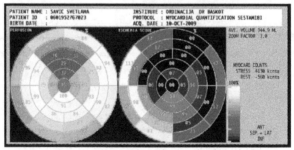

quantification of perfusion by Stierner
- segments quantification 10/10/2009

Radonuclide ventriculography for evaluating global ejection fraction Performed before and after HBO = EPO therapy

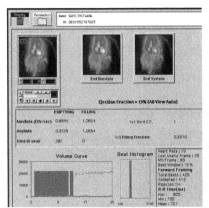

radionuclide ventriculography (RNV)
performed 07.17. 2009 before therapy

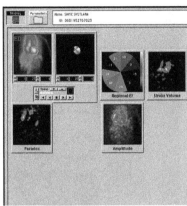

radionuclide ventriculography (RNV)
regional ejection fraction

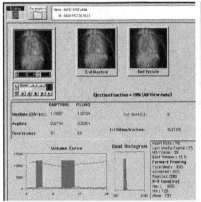

radionuclide ventriculography (RNV)
performed 10.12.2009 after therapy

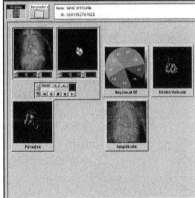

radionuclide ventriculography (RNV)
regional ejection fraction

Case report 2. Male with non-ischemic heart failure

SPECT scan performed before HBO = EPO therapy

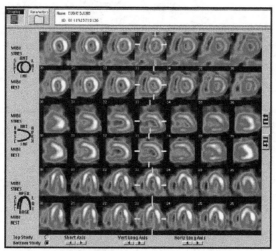

SPECT MPI performed 13.01.2011
Scan pattern - dilatative myocardiopathy
non-ischemic type

Radionuclide venticulography performed before and after HBO = EPO therapy when we seen
the greatest increase of LVEF with improve wall motion and regional kinetics

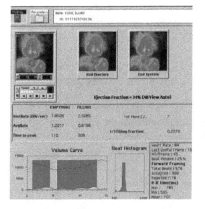
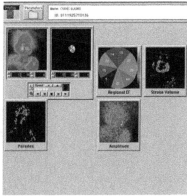

RNV with global and regional ejection fraction performed 01.17. 2011 – before therapy

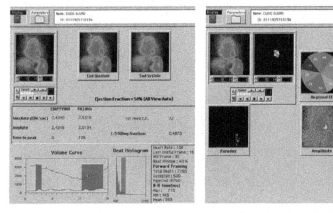

RNV with global and regional ejection fraction performed 03.23. 2011 – after therapy

Summary

The field of cardiovascular imaging is changing. In one hand, myocardial perfusion imaging is a well/established clinical technique for the diagnostic and prognostic workup of coronary artery disease. It has been the mainstay of nuclear cardiology for decades. On the other hand, several alternative imaging methodologies for noninvasive functional assessment of ischemic heart disease have emerged, and noninvasive coronary angiography is becoming a clinical reality. Nuclear imaging technology has progressed significantly toward higher sensitivity and resolution, and novel, highly specific radiotracers have been introduced. These developments are indicator of steady evolution of nuclear cardiology beyond the assessment of myocardial perfusion and toward characterization of biologic events on the tissue level. It is hoped that radiotracers techniques, with their unique translational potential and their superior detection sensitivity, will take a leading role in personalized cardiovascular medicine, in which therapeutic and/or preventive strategies are based on individual disease biology. The value of more specific imaging targets, which are increasingly entering clinical practice. This includes imaging of heart failure, absolute quantification of myocardial blood flow, imaging of myocardial metabolism, and imaging of the cardiac autonomic nervous system.

The goal of this chapter is to provide the reader with a comprehensive overview of the most recent development in nuclear cardiology, in the era of interventional cardiology. It is hoped that the reader, after going through this article, will share the enthusiasm of the author for this discipline, which holds the potential to be a key component in the new paradigm of early detection coronary artery disease for indication for interventional cardiology, as well as assessment new therapeutic effect (HBO + EPO) of heart failure.

Author details

Branislav Baskot[1], Igor Ivanov[2], Dragan Kovacevic[2], Slobodan Obradovic[3], Nenad Ratkovic[3] and Miodrag Zivkovic[4]

1 Private "Clinic Dr Baskot", Belgrade, Serbia

2 Institute for Cardiovascular Disease Sremska Kamenica, Serbia

3 Clinic for Urgent Medicine, Medical Military Academy, Belgrade, Serbia

4 HBO Medical Center, Medical Practice for Hyperbaric Oxygenation Therapy, Belgrade, Serbia

References

[1] ACC/AHA/ASNC Guidelines for the Clinical Use of Cardiac Radionuclide Imaging. A Report of the American College of Cardiology/American Heart Association Task Force on Practice Guidelines (ACC/AHA/ASNC Committee to Revise the 1995 Guidelines for the Clinical Use of cardiac Radionuclide Imaging). Journal of the American Coll Cardiol October. 1. 2003. ACC/AHA/ASNC Practice Guidelines 01–69.

[2] Branislav Baskot: Nuclear cardiology - determination of culprit lesion. Belgrade: Andrejevic foundation; 2006.

[3] Garry V. Heller, Robert C. Hendel: Nuclear Cardiology – practical application 259-71 The McGroaw-Hill Companies, Inc. 2004

[4] Masud H. Khandaker, Tod D. Miller, Panithaya Chateronthaitawee, J. Wells Askew, David O. Hodge, Raymond J. Gibbons: Stress single photon emission computed tomography for detection of coronary artery disease and risk stratification of asymptomatic patients at moderate risk. Journal of Nuclear Cardiology Vol 16, No 4;516-23 July/August 2009

[5] Shaw LJ, Hendel R., Borges-Neto S. Lauer MS: Prognostic value of normal exercise and adenosine (99m) Tc-tetrofosmine SPECT imaging; results from the multicenter registry of 4,728 patients. J Nucl Med 44: 134, 2003

[6] Baskot B, Rafajlovski S, Ristić-Angelkov A, Obradović S, Gligić B, Orozović V, Agbaba N.: Study of efficacy and safety of pharmacological stress tests in nuclear cardiology. Vojnosanit Pregl. 2009 Mar;66(3):193-8. Serbian.

[7] Michael I. Miyamoto, Sharon L. Vernicoto, Haresh Majmundar, Gregory S. Thomas: Pharmacological stress myocardial perfusion imaging: A practical approach. Journal of Nuclear Cardiology 2007; vol 14 No 2, 250-55

[8] Georg A. Beller: Compliance with appropriate use criteria for cardiac radionuclide imaging. Journal of Nuclear Cardiology vol 17; No 2;165-67 March/April 2010

[9] Tim J.F., Johannes C. Kelder, Herbert W.M. Plokker, J. Fred Verzijlbergen, Norbert M. van Hemel: Myocardial perfusion SPECT identifies patients with left bundle branch block patterns at high risk for future cardiac events. Journal of Nuclear Cardiology vol 17; No 2;216-24 March/April 2010

[10] Georg A. Beller; Implications of randomized studies of medical therapy vs revascularization for reducing rising costs of helth care. Journal of Nuclear Cradiology vol 16. No 4;483-85 July/August 2009

[11] American Heart Association Writing Group on Myocardial Segmentation and Registration for Cardiac Imaging. Standardized myocardial segmentation and nomenclature for tomographic imaging of the heart: A statement for healthcare professionals from the Cardiac Imaging Committee of the Council on Clinical Cardiology of the American Heart Association. Circulation 2002; 105:539–42.

[12] Gary V. Heller, Robert C. Hendel.: Nuclear Cardiology Practical Applications. McGraw-Hill medical Publishing divison. The McGraw-Hill Companies, Inc. Copyright 2004; 193-243

[13] Udelson JE., Beshansky JR., Ballin DS.: Myocardial perfusion imaging for evaluation and triage of patients with suspected acute cardiac ischemia: a randomized controlled trial. JAMA 2002; 288:2693-2700

[14] Baskot B., Jankovic Z., Obradovic S., Rusovic S., Orozovic V., Gligic B., Jung R., Ivanovic V., Pavlovic M., Ratkovic N.,: Diagnostic significance of myocardial perfusion scintigraphy in identification and localization of culprit lesions in patients undergoing elective PTCA. VSP vol 65; No 2 (158-62) ; 2008

[15] Leslee J Shaw, Allen Taylor, Paolo Raggi, Daniel S Berman: Role of noninvasive imaging in asymptomatic high/risk patients. J Nucl Cardiol 2006; vol 13 No2(156-62).

[16] AN Clarc, GA Beller: The present role of nuclear cardiology in clinical practice. The quarterly journal of Nuclear Medicine and Molecular Imaging. vol. 49 No 1(43-58) March 2005.

[17] Barry L. Zaret, George A. Beller: Clinical Nuclear Cardiology; state of the art and future directions. Elsevier Mosby. 2005.

[18] Vasken Dilsizian, Jagat Narula; Atlas of Nuclear Cardiology – second edition. Current medicine LLC 2006.

[19] Baskot B, Zivković M, Tepić S, Obradović S.: Evaluation of the therapeutic effect of hyperbaric oxygenation and erithropoietin in the treatment of chronic heart failure using myocardial perfusion scintigraphy G/SPECT. Vojnosanit Pregl. 2009 May;66(5): 399-402.

[20] Zivkovic Miodrag: Guide for Hyperbaric Medicine. Serbian Health Organization, Belgrade, Serbia. - 2010.

[21] Zivkovic M., Todorovic V., Tepic S., Jakovljevic V. Synergistic application of hyperbaric oxygenation therapy and erythropoietin in treatment of ch ronic heart failure. Medical review, No. 1-2, pp. 19/24. Novi Sad Serbia, 2007

Permissions

The contributors of this book come from diverse backgrounds, making this book a truly international effort. This book will bring forth new frontiers with its revolutionizing research information and detailed analysis of the nascent developments around the world.

We would like to thank Branislav G. Baskot MD PhD, for lending his expertise to make the book truly unique. He has played a crucial role in the development of this book. Without his invaluable contribution this book wouldn't have been possible. He has made vital efforts to compile up to date information on the varied aspects of this subject to make this book a valuable addition to the collection of many professionals and students.

This book was conceptualized with the vision of imparting up-to-date information and advanced data in this field. To ensure the same, a matchless editorial board was set up. Every individual on the board went through rigorous rounds of assessment to prove their worth. After which they invested a large part of their time researching and compiling the most relevant data for our readers. Conferences and sessions were held from time to time between the editorial board and the contributing authors to present the data in the most comprehensible form. The editorial team has worked tirelessly to provide valuable and valid information to help people across the globe.

Every chapter published in this book has been scrutinized by our experts. Their significance has been extensively debated. The topics covered herein carry significant findings which will fuel the growth of the discipline. They may even be implemented as practical applications or may be referred to as a beginning point for another development. Chapters in this book were first published by InTech; hereby published with permission under the Creative Commons Attribution License or equivalent.

The editorial board has been involved in producing this book since its inception. They have spent rigorous hours researching and exploring the diverse topics which have resulted in the successful publishing of this book. They have passed on their knowledge of decades through this book. To expedite this challenging task, the publisher supported the team at every step. A small team of assistant editors was also appointed to further simplify the editing procedure and attain best results for the readers.

Our editorial team has been hand-picked from every corner of the world. Their multi-ethnicity adds dynamic inputs to the discussions which result in innovative outcomes. These outcomes are then further discussed with the researchers and contributors who give their valuable feedback and opinion regarding the same. The feedback is then collaborated with the researches and they are edited in a comprehensive manner to aid the understanding of the subject.

Apart from the editorial board, the designing team has also invested a significant amount of their time in understanding the subject and creating the most relevant covers. They scrutinized every image to scout for the most suitable representation of the subject and create an appropriate cover for the book.

The publishing team has been involved in this book since its early stages. They were actively engaged in every process, be it collecting the data, connecting with the contributors or procuring relevant information. The team has been an ardent support to the editorial, designing and production team. Their endless efforts to recruit the best for this project, has resulted in the accomplishment of this book. They are a veteran in the field of academics and their pool of knowledge is as vast as their experience in printing. Their expertise and guidance has proved useful at every step. Their uncompromising quality standards have made this book an exceptional effort. Their encouragement from time to time has been an inspiration for everyone.

The publisher and the editorial board hope that this book will prove to be a valuable piece of knowledge for researchers, students, practitioners and scholars across the globe.

List of Contributors

Catarina Ramos and Teresa Pinheiro
IST/ITN Instituto Superior Técnico, Universidade Técnica de Lisboa, Sacavém, Portugal

Patrícia Napoleão
Unidade de Biologia Microvascular e Inflamação, Instituto de Medicina Molecular, Faculdade de Medicina da Universidade de Lisboa, Lisboa, Portugal

Rui Cruz Ferreira, Cristina Fondinho and Mafalda Selas
Serviço Cardiologia, Hospital Santa Marta, Centro Hospitalar Lisboa Central, Lisboa, Portugal

Miguel Mota Carmo and Ana Maria Crespo
Centro de Estudos de Doenças Crónicas, Faculdade de Ciências Médicas, Universidade Nova de Lisboa & Serviço Cardiologia, Hospital Santa Marta Centro Hospitalar Lisboa Central, Lisboa, Portugal

Massimo Cocchi
"Paolo Sotgiu" Institute for research in Quantitative & Quantum Psychiatry & Cardiology, L.U.de.S University, Lugano, Switzerland
Department of Medical Veterinary Sciences, University of Bologna, Italy

Giovanni Lercker
DISA, University of Bologna, Italy

Karthikeyan Ananthasubramaniam and Sabha Bhatti
Henry Ford Hospital, Heart and Vascular Institute, Detroit MI, USA

Abdul Hakeem
William Beaumont Hospital Royal Oak MI, USA

Jasmin Čaluk
BH Heart Center, Department of interventional cardiology, Tuzla, Bosnia and Herzegovina

Maurizio Turiel and Luigi Gianturco
Cardiology Unit, IRCCS Galeazzi Orthopedic Institute, Department of Biomedical Sciences for Health, University of Milan, Milan, Italy

Vincenzo Gianturco
Department of Cardiovascular, Respiratory, Nephrological, Anesthesiological and Geriatrics Sciences, Sapienza University of Rome, Italy

Bruno Dino Bodini
Rehabilitation Unit, IRCCS Galeazzi Orthopedic Institute, Italy

G.J. Pelgrim and R. Vliegenthart
Department of Radiology, University of Groningen, University Medical Center Groningen, Groningen, Netherlands
Center for Medical Imaging – North East Netherlands, University of Groningen, University Medical Center Groningen, Groningen, Netherlands

M. Oudkerk
Center for Medical Imaging – North East Netherlands, University of Groningen, University Medical Center Groningen, Groningen, Netherlands

Takao Hasegawa and Kenei Shimada
Department of Internal Medicine and Cardiology, Osaka City University Graduate School of Medicine, Abeno-ku, Osaka, Japan

Ri-ichiro Kakihara
Department of Cardiology, Private Kakihara Clinic, Toyohashi, Japan

Bong Gun Song
Cardiovascular Imaging Center, Cardiac and Vascular Center, Konkuk University Medical Center, Republic of Korea

Branislav Baskot
Private "Clinic Dr Baskot", Belgrade, Serbia

Igor Ivanov and Dragan Kovacevic
Institute for Cardiovascular Disease Sremska Kamenica, Serbia

Slobodan Obradovic and Nenad Ratkovic
Clinic for Urgent Medicine, Medical Military Academy, Belgrade, Serbia

Miodrag Zivkovic
HBO Medical Center, Medical Practice for Hyperbaric Oxygenation Therapy, Belgrade, Serbia

Printed in the USA
CPSIA information can be obtained
at www.ICGtesting.com
JSHW011420221024
72173JS00004B/606